Now It's Mary's Turn

Year One

Mary E. Clark
Foreword by Dr. Irit Gat, Ph.D.

This book is dedicated to my circle of friends,
family and teachers without whose unconditional love
and encouragement, "Year One," the book
and year one after weight loss surgery
would have been a much harder journey.

Travis, Nick, Damien, Adrian, Grace, Sadie, Zoe,
Mom & Dad, Anne, Nini, Dr. John Yadegar and Dr. Irit Gat,
I love you and I'm grateful.

Foreword

Reading "Now It's Mary's Turn – Year One," is like having a copy of her personal journal. Perhaps I feel this way because I remember what she was going through at the time.

Mary and I met in 2009 when she began working with the bariatric surgical program I'd been with for the past four years. We clicked immediately. I was energized by her love for the patients and eagerness to create more learning opportunities for them. We collaborated on multiple projects and our friendship developed along the way.

In 2011, when Mary told me she decided to have surgery, I remember telling her, "You're going to do great. You know so much about the surgery already, and we're all here for you."

Then only a few months into her first year, a time when most patients are still adjusting to the physical aspects of the surgery and focusing on all the changes that accompany it, Mary's life was turned upside down. I remember thinking how difficult it would be to go through a gut-wrenching divorce and be successful the first year after weight loss surgery. Understandably for some, it would be one or the other. But for Mary, one or the other was not an option.

She did what I've seen her do so many times before. She assessed the situation and figured it out. I remember suggesting that she look into therapy, only to hear her response, "Oh I did, but my insurance plan can only see me 3-4 times per year. So I'm doing it myself." Then she told me about the books, videos and other resources she had been diving into. There were difficult moments for sure, and they rest between the lines of each story in "Year One" as Mary questions what she thought she knew about bariatric surgery and life. But something told me, although I suspected she had a long road ahead, she'd be okay.

"We have so many memories, hurts, sorrows and failures, all associated with our lives of obesity. And perhaps we occasionally used our obesity to protect us from people, activities, experiences and life. Sometimes it seems like the greater work after weight loss surgery is not exercising, eating right or taking supplements, but working on what's inside. Healing everything we have associated with obesity, making peace with our past lives. And now, accepting and making peace with our new lives in these healthier bodies."

Because of her background, Mary is definitely all about patients following their surgeon's instructions for nutrition, exercise, vitamins, medical follow-up, and support. And while she does explore familiar bariatric surgery topics, the reader benefits from Mary's uncommon insight as a post-op patient, weight loss surgery educator and advocate, and a woman figuring out how to care for her children and herself during a painful divorce. It is because of this trifecta and Mary's steadfast determination to figure it out, that she provides her reader with a unique experience of life after weight loss surgery. As her world is collapsing and her health simultaneously restored, she takes courageous steps to create a new life.

"My doctor can't see it. Either can a spouse, partner, sister, boyfriend or best friend. Even when you try to explain what you're feeling, thinking and how much you've changed. You're the only one who really knows how much. I'm the only one who knows to what degree I've changed my thinking, reacting, my self-talk. I'm the only one who's aware of every thought I have and every decision I make. Only I know if I'm really eating and exercising the way I should, and when I'm not- only I know the reason WHY and that's only if I pay attention to WHY."

"Now It's Mary's Turn – Year One," is not just a book for those considering bariatric surgery or the newly operated, but it also serves those who want to rediscover their motivation and reclaim their weight loss journey.

-Dr. Irit Gat, Ph.D.

Author's Note

About three weeks before I had weight loss surgery in May, 2011, I started a blog, "Now It's Mary's Turn." I wanted to share my story publicly because I believed I offered a unique perspective since I'd been working in bariatric surgery for ten years. What I didn't know at the time was how drastically my headline was about to change:

"Weight loss surgery educator achieves picture-perfect success as a direct result of her extensive knowledge and experience in the field!"

instead I got...

"Even ten years as a weight loss surgery educator and working with top experts in the field, couldn't prepare Mary for what happened during her first year after surgery."

It's definitely not the story I had planned.

After my surgery I had a few blissful months of weight loss, then all hell broke loose.

On September 26, 2011, about two weeks into my life falling apart, I wrote:

"If you're in the pre-op stage, you're going for tests...it's easy to get caught up in the physical stuff and think that the mental stuff will just work itself out after surgery. But you must put the work into it and prepare now. How will you handle the stress? And choose your exercise now. Cultivate your group of supporting and loving friends and family, now. Put just as much effort into these areas as you do choosing the perfect protein powder and ordering vitamins. You never know how soon after surgery you're going to need them."

I was writing to myself.

I'm the one who…
needed to know how to handle the stress,
needed to find the exercise that would help me work out my frustration and sadness,
needed the support of loving friends and family.

I believe in weight loss surgery, but it's only a tool. Self-control, willpower and stress management techniques aren't implanted during surgery.

The biggest work after weight loss surgery is within yourself.

If you're preparing for surgery or had it recently, I hope the following stories encourage, inspire and motivate you to plan for life beyond protein shakes, vitamins, and the scale.

If you're further out from surgery and dealing with a plateau or regain, I hope these stories remind you of the courage you've already demonstrated, and how with a heart and mindset shift you can live the life you dreamed of before you had surgery.

Sitting here five years later, I can see how my weight loss surgery journey was absolutely the one I needed to go through. It had all the lessons I needed to learn so I could finally get to this place. The happiest, healthiest and most at peace I've ever been in my life.

Sweetheart, I want this for you too.

~Mary

One more thing.

If you visit maryeclark.com, receive my weekly emails or connect with me on social media, you may notice that my writing style and voice from 2011-2012 is different. When I prepared "Year One" for you, I chose minimal editing because I wanted the stories to remain true to what I was thinking and feeling during my first year of weight loss surgery and at the end of my marriage. This is who I was then.

We're keeping it real here.

Okay, go ahead and dive in now!

Table of Contents

Pre-Op

"I really have tried so hard but I can't do it this time. My body can't take anymore suffering and neither can I."

"I may not even need my diabetes medication two weeks from now…but what if something's wrong with my lab work and I can't have surgery next week?"

"They were talking about the years of pain, sadness, and embarrassment, that with the surgery would finally be over."

3-6 Months

19 - My brain can't keep up with my body.
Pages 72 - 73

"These are real feelings you need to be ready for. It takes time to process all the physical, mental and emotional changes you go through."

20 - You never know how soon you'll need this.
Pages 74 - 76

"At 4-months post-op, there are things I could eat to deal with the stress, but I'm not. I won't say I'm handling this stressful time perfectly, but better than I would have before surgery."

21 - I'm trying not to miss a thing.
Pages 77 - 79

"To not have your weight be an obstacle to something as simple as buying a tin of tea? These moments come around more often and I try not to miss them."

22 - Waiting for the other shoe to drop.
Pages 80 - 83

"I'm not waking up every morning focused on my weight. I wake up and live without the burden of obesity. It used to consume my life."

23 - Here's the proof.
Pages 84 - 87

"It's even greater validation that I made the right decision to have surgery and make my life better in every way."

29 - Human nature.
Pages 111 - 115

"It took me months to even admit that my overeating was emotional, my way of coping. And when life gets rough there are days I still want to turn to food to numb the pain."

30 - I stopped exercising.
Pages 116 - 119

"I couldn't bring myself to do any exercise for five days straight. I felt defeated and I wasn't exercising at all."

9-12 Months

31 - Who's in your circle?
Pages 120 - 123

"We must find the courage to say, "This was my choice…I'm the only one who has to live in this body and this is how I chose to improve my life.""

32 - You're building a house.
Pages 124 - 128

"It's my responsibility to utilize all the tools. If I leave out strong support circles or consistent exercise, my long-term success is diminished."

33 - The phantom of fat.
Pages 129 - 132

"The greater work after weight loss surgery is making peace with our past lives. And now, accepting and making peace with our new lives in these healthier bodies."

39 - Backup plan activated.
Pages 150 - 151

"The huge black and blue bruise across my foot reminds me how I haven't been able to wear a shoe for the last week. Things happen, so we have to have backup plans."

40 - Year One. My surgery anniversary.
Pages 152 - 160

"Before surgery how many days did I wake up wishing I wasn't obese, praying for the strength to stick with a diet and exercise plan, pleading with God to not let my diabetes or other conditions get any worse. SEVEN days a week. Since surgery, how many days have I felt this way? ZERO."

- 1 -

Why I've Decided to Have Weight Loss Surgery
May 10

I'm actually a very private person. So to make the decision to write openly about my sad, life-long struggle with weight is something I never thought I would do, but here I am.

My perspective on weight and weight loss surgery is somewhat different because I've worked in the bariatric surgery field for 10 years. I believe in it. I know the risks and benefits, the good, the bad, the ugly and the truly beautiful. I've been inside the operating room watching the surgery happen. I've seen the patients go from barely being able to go for a walk in the park to skydiving.

So how did I get here?

Together, my husband and I have 5 kids. I came into our marriage with two, he had one, and then we had two more.

I've given birth to BIG babies:

Travis: 10.6 lbs.
Nick: 12.10 lbs.
Adrian: 13 lbs. (C-section 2 weeks early)
Grace: 12 lbs. (C-section 1 month early to avoid a 15-pound baby!)

I had gestational diabetes with all of them. With proper eating and lots of exercise I lost the baby weight after each of the first three. But after my daughter was born in 1998, it didn't happen.

Every month I started a new diet, exercised when I could, and for a while that was pretty regular. I maintained a size 14 for about seven years, and then moved up to size 16 for about two years, and for the last two years an 18 or 20. What else have I worn for the past two years?

Diabetes.

My diabetes diagnosis came in early 2010 following my Rheumatoid Arthritis diagnosis in 2004, Fibromyalgia and liver disease (from the enormous amounts of medications I was taking) in 2005, and Hashimoto's Disease in 2009. By late 2010 I was injecting insulin. With my BMI at 40 and diabetes, I was a perfect candidate for weight loss surgery. I made the decision to move forward only to learn that my husband's employer chose not to cover bariatric surgery under their PPO plan. The irony, right? Especially since he worked for a hospital. It was depressing, to say the least.

I made a conscious effort to exercise and eat healthier. But then life happened as it always has and always does.

Grandchildren are born, 92 year-old aunts without their own children to care for them break their hips and need help, work gets really busy, and so on and so on.

So my healthy habits fell by the way side again, as I was dashing around trying to take care of everybody else.

Sound familiar?

I was taking care of everybody except myself. I felt helpless and that's not me. My husband and I chose to go with an HMO for 2011. I never had an HMO before, but it was my only option to get bariatric surgery covered. It turned out to be the best decision we ever made about our healthcare.

So far, the pre-op process has been very smooth. I had my final test last week. The results came in today and all looks well. I'm scheduled for surgery on May 23rd. It hit me hard today when I got the call about the last test being okay. I almost started crying. It's really very emotional.

It's really happening!

My daughter hugged me in the middle of Target, then we stocked up on lots of sugar-free Jello and fat-free/sugar-free pudding!

I work with the surgeon who will perform my surgery. I'm asked if that will be strange to have him do my surgery, but my answer is, "No." He's a professional, wonderful, and I trust him completely.

Although I've been around weight loss surgery for a long time, when it's happening to you it's completely different!

I've taught pre and post-op classes, moderated support groups, coached patients preparing for surgery, educated physicians about the procedures, attended the annual conferences for the American Society of Metabolic and Bariatric Surgery, worked with some of the best teams developing education programs, been privy to the latest research and outcome studies, and yet I still feel like a fish out of water and that I want to read everything all over again because this time it's happening to ME!

So I'm less than two weeks away from surgery and yes, I'm a little nervous. But when I think about being off my diabetes medications and no longer injecting insulin, the nervousness subsides. I want to do all the things my patients tell me about in their success stories.

Play with my kids and my granddaughter.
Wear a sundress at the beach.
Ride a bike comfortably.
Hike with my son.
Shop in regular stores.
Not feel like people are thinking less of me because of my weight.

I'm so tired of waking up every morning having my first thoughts be about my weight and my failing health. Sometimes when I feel the burning, tingling sensations in my feet from diabetes, I wonder if I'll make it to my 60s. I wonder if they'll find a cure for diabetes before that. I think my husband will outlive me. I really have tried so hard and I've lost the weight on my own many times before, but I can't do it this time.

I can't do it this time. My body can't take anymore suffering and neither can I.

I told my surgeon that if weight loss surgery did nothing else but take away my diabetes and my need for insulin injections, I would still do it. I see the looks on my kids' faces when they walk into a room and I'm injecting insulin into my stomach. I see the look on my husband's face when I'm desperately thirsty almost to the point of panic.

I feel like I've done everything I can do and surgery is what MUST be done to save my life.

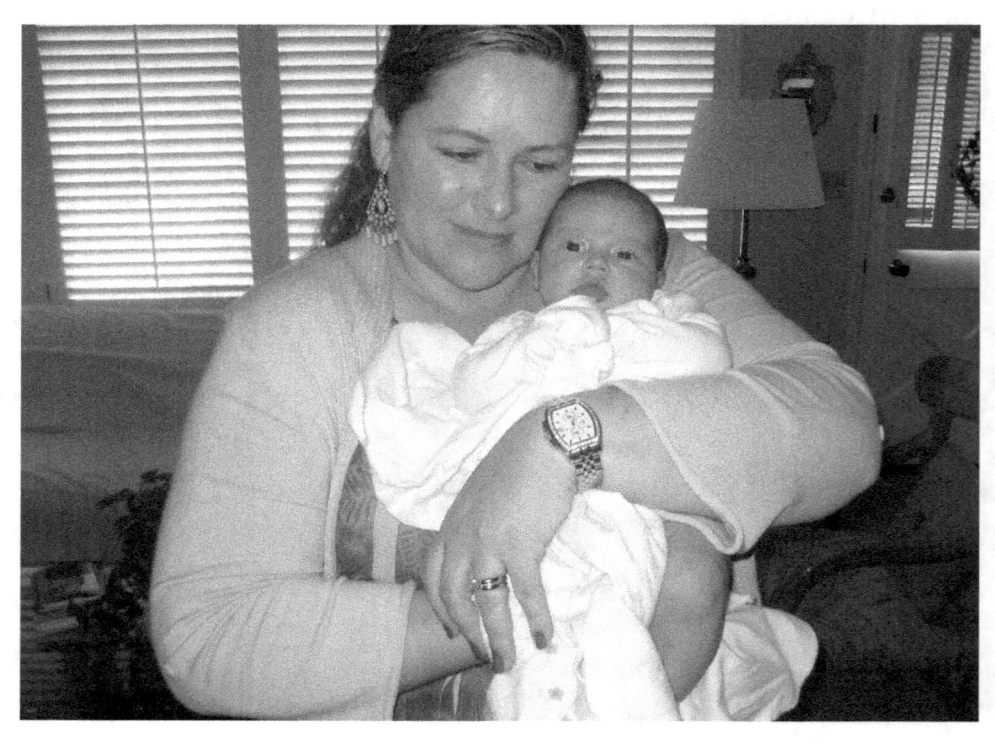

- 2 -

One Week Until Surgery
May 16

I imagine this is normal, but the surgery enters into my mind almost all the time now. I continue with my normal activities at work and at home, but everything reminds me of the changes coming. I talk about the actual hospital stay quite simply, "Oh, I need a robe," and I tell my husband, "Honey, there will be quite a bit of traffic driving up." Yes, it's all very matter-of-fact. But am I trying to avoid what's really going on in my head?

WOW! THERE ARE BIG CHANGES COMING!

And although I've heard many patients tell me about their experiences, I'm wondering what the changes really feel like. I know there's physical and emotional changes, the impact on my family, the impact on my health, the impact on my life! I filled my diabetes medications last week and I thought, "I may not even need these two weeks from now!" I need to go in for my pre-op labs today and there is still that little voice inside that says, "What if something's wrong with my lab work and I can't have surgery next week?"

I've worked in bariatric surgery for more than ten years, I've seen it happen. A patient catches a cold, a late test result comes back positive and the surgeon needs another test. A snowstorm. Okay, it's May in Southern California so that's unlikely.

Or are these thoughts of nervousness?

Again, I'm telling myself this is all normal, as with any big event in one's life, there are nerves and excitement involved. My faith in God tells me all will be well this week and my surgery will take place next Monday as scheduled.

Breathe, Mary. Breathe.

- 3 -

5 Days Until Surgery
May 18

I hope I'm five days away. I had to have a stress-echocardiogram on Monday and I'm waiting on the results. I've never personally understood the anxiety this very situation has caused for so many patients until right now. I'm learning so much already.

I'm recalling how many patients I've talked to in situations just like this. They're in tears, telling me how long they've waited to have surgery. Now I know what they were truly talking about. It wasn't just about the time it had taken them to prepare for the actual surgery. They were talking about the years and years of pain, sadness, embarrassment, isolation, depression, feelings of failure, that they believed with the surgery would finally be over or on their way to being over.

Weight loss surgery represents hope, a way to live again and enjoy life.

For some, who've never been a normal weight, it will be the very first time. And now I understand why so many patients celebrate their surgery date as their new birthday. My surgery date happens to be on my son Adrian's birthday, and the day before my son Nick's birthday. We'll celebrate three birthdays now!

So wish me luck that this last test comes out okay and that my surgery date stays as scheduled.

Yes, Tom Petty, the waiting is the hardest part.

- 4 -

Last Test Is Negative - The Surgery Is On!
May 18

just got the news. The last test is negative and this is really happening. I jumped up and down hugging my daughter in Target. I called my other kids and e-mailed a few people who all said, "We told you it would all workout!" Deep down inside I knew it would too, but it's fantastic to have the final confirmation that it's a go!

Yesterday I spoke with a patient, about a year out from surgery. She looks amazing. She told me she looks at herself in the mirror now and says, "You're hot!" I love that! And even though I hope I'll feel like that about myself someday, it doesn't even seem real. When I told her I was having surgery she told me:

"I got my walking started in the hospital, when the nurses said I could stop, I kept going!"

"I went for a walk on Santa Monica Pier right after I was

discharged from the hospital."

"As soon as the doctor gave me the okay, I started swimming, and kept swimming every day."

"I followed all of his directions, I ate what he said to eat. I drank what he said to drink. I took care of myself."

I remember seeing this patient about 3 months after surgery. Her transformation was incredible because she'd been swimming daily. Her body was shrinking in all areas. When you see her now, after more than 150 pounds, her arms are toned, tummy nearly flat and her legs are in great shape. She was recently promoted at work and is confident that her new energy, vitality, and health contributed to this latest success.

So, my husband and Grace will go with me on Monday. My surgery will begin at 9:30 a.m. and should be over in about two hours. We're taking pictures, and as soon as I can I'll document how it went and how I'm feeling.

Until then, I have a fun weekend of liquids and uh, cleaning out my system.

Thanks for your well wishes, support, and prayers!

- 5 -

We Did It
May 27

I have to say WE, because this could not have happened without the team! My husband, kids, and my mom and sister who took my sons out for their birthdays while I was in the hospital. Thank you to my phenomenal surgeon. Yes, he's as great as all the patients say he is. It's different seeing him from the patient's side. He's pretty close to perfect.

I got home yesterday after staying an extra night due to a fever, which I tend to get after I have surgery.

So how was it? I'm going to give you the details or at least most of them. Monday, the day of surgery, it hurt. Not my stomach, but actually my back. Apparently I did not get myself into the most comfortable position before anesthesia and my back didn't do well, and I don't have back problems.

My friend stayed with me Monday night and helped me on

my walks. I do recommend having someone stay with you, at least the first night. You're not moving around very well and it's good to have someone nearby. I also recommend you limit your visitors the first day. I wasn't really in the mood to chat, visit, or even talk on the phone. So plan on that and tell everyone before you go to the hospital not to visit or even call the first day.

By Tuesday the back pain was much better and I still had no stomach pain. I started alternating the protein shake and water, and everything went down really well. The drain bothered me, though. It didn't hurt, but it was just hanging there and pulled a little bit. None of the incisions hurt, thank goodness!

Walking got easier and easier, and the catheter came out. Going to the bathroom was fine. It's much better to have visitors and phone calls on the day after surgery. It's really important to keep track of the protein and water on the form the nurse gives you. Now that I mention the nurses, THANK YOU! You were all awesome and took such good care of me. I couldn't have asked for a better hospital stay.

Wednesday morning the drain came out. HALLELUJAH! It did feel a little weird when my surgeon took it out, but he told me to expect that. It was sort of like this thing is coiled up in your stomach and when he pulls on it it's moving through you. Okay, I had to tell you that, but it didn't hurt.

I need to finish up the surgery adventure tomorrow. I'm going to take a short nap and then heading out with Grace to see GLEE in concert at the HONDA center. Yes, I'm feeling that good! I even called ahead and got their okay to bring my protein shake and water with me because I had surgery. They were great about it.

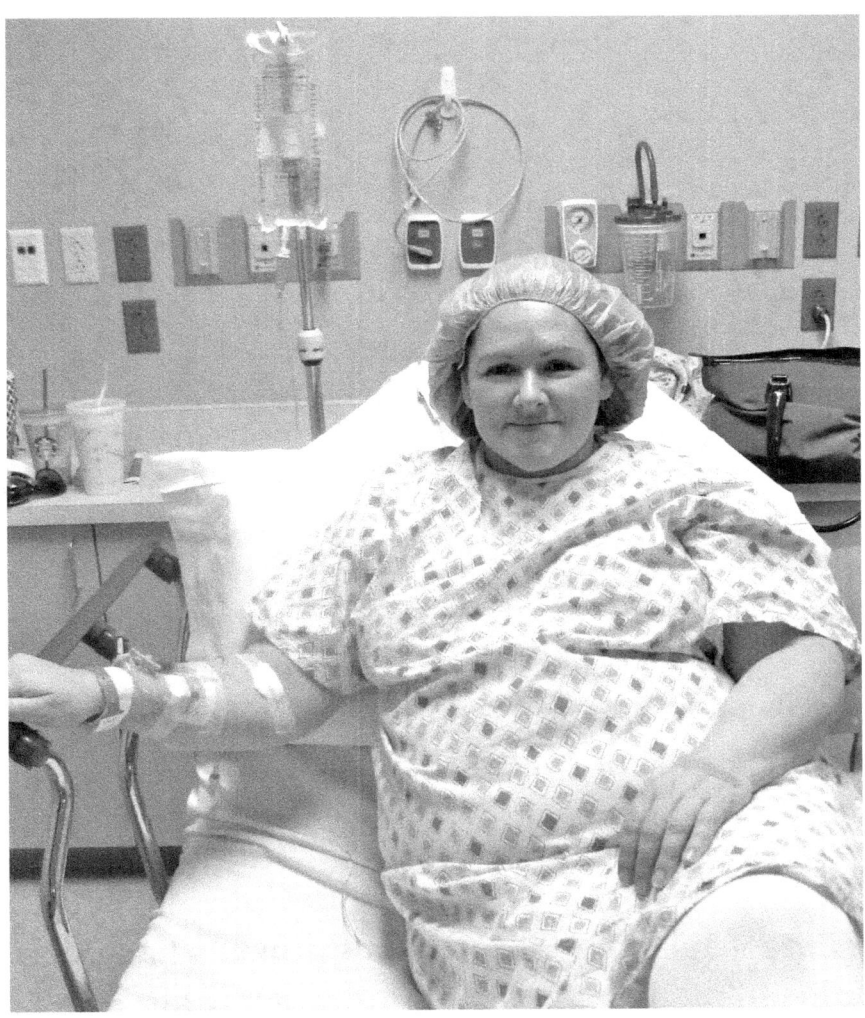

- 6 -

We Did It (Part 2)
May 28

I'm back! On Wednesday I was running a temperature of about 101.5 and my potassium was low, so my surgeon decided to keep me another night. The protein and water were going down and staying down just fine. The nurse said my input (protein and water) matched my output (urine) almost exactly. Everything was moving just fine. I kept walking and tried to nap when I could. Yes, the staff was wonderful, but in being wonderful they have to take vitals and check on you as scheduled, so that means you don't really get much solid sleep.

My surgeon said by day two, some patients have buyer's remorse, regretting they had surgery. I have to admit that my back hurt bad enough on the day of surgery that I asked myself, "What did I do?" Thankfully that passed by Tuesday morning. But I never regretted the actual surgery.

By Thursday I was ready to go home! My fever was gone

and I was just finishing up my potassium through the IV. I got my discharge instructions and eating plan for the next two weeks. My husband drove up from work in Long Beach to pick us up. Grace stayed with my lovely friend who lives near the hospital so she could be near me. I don't know if I mentioned that I had surgery 85 miles away from home! My surgeon emphasizes to patients who live more than 30 minutes away, to walk every thirty minutes on the drive home and I did. It was great to get home and SLEEP IN MY OWN BED!

Friday I felt fine. I used the timer on my phone to alternate water and protein every 10 minutes because it's easy to forget to drink. I've always been a water drinker and that makes drinking water pretty easy for me. I've always had a water bottle with me.

But for protein, well you're just not hungry, ever! So this is important; use a timer or some kind of reminder to get in your protein and water, otherwise you won't feel so good. Friday evening, my husband drove us to the HONDA Center in Anaheim for the GLEE concert. I walked two large flights of stairs to get to our seats and had no problem standing during the show and even danced a bit! I didn't take a nap Friday although I had planned on it, but I still made it. I was pretty tired when I got home though.

Saturday I spent the day with my family at my mom's house. When I got there my mom said she hadn't eaten lunch yet so I made her a sandwich. This was the first food I prepared after surgery and I wondered how it would be knowing I couldn't eat. No problem. Really. This has to be because I'm not hungry. I played with my granddaughter although it was hard not to pick her up, but we managed.

For dinner I ordered pizza from our favorite neighborhood place, and watched my family enjoy it. It smelled great, looked yummy, but I was still okay. My granddaughter and I shared Jello, my first food since surgery, and it went down just fine. That night I had sugar-free/fat-free cheesecake pudding and had no problems.

Sunday I went grocery shopping. I have a family and they still eat. I felt great, and although the fresh baked bread smelled really good, I was able to select a loaf knowing I would not be eating it. I went home and made chili beans and chicken soup. My daughter was on-hand for taste testing, although I sampled the chicken soup broth. I enjoyed the cooking, but still had no hunger. I took a walk in the evening and then enjoyed homemade chicken broth with my family. Later I had a sugar-free popsicle. It tasted great and again no issues.

I'm getting down 5-6, 16-ounce bottles of water daily, half with Crystal Light. I was already a water drinker so perhaps this is already a habit for me. But I've heard so many patients in the past say they couldn't get all the water down. I'm not having any issues with water. I'm also consuming three protein shakes each day with 30-40 grams of protein in each. And then I'll have a popsicle, some broth or pudding.

I haven't weighed myself yet. There's no particular reason why. Okay, maybe I'm just nervous. I bought a new scale about a month ago. My surgeon said to check it just once a week. I should probably weigh myself later today since surgery was a week ago. My family says my tummy looks smaller and I see the difference a little too. Okay, I see it more than a little. But I'm reserved in getting excited. We've all done the diets and you get excited when you see some results, no matter how small. But very often, those results were short-lived.

Knowing that these results are life-long, if I follow all the guidelines, is something I have not wrapped my head around yet. My daughter took my measurements the night before surgery. I'll ask her to measure me again today and then weekly. I'm thinking I'll probably measure success by inches instead of pounds. Why? Honestly, the numbers on the scale, at least right now, still scare me. Maybe I'll get there, one day.

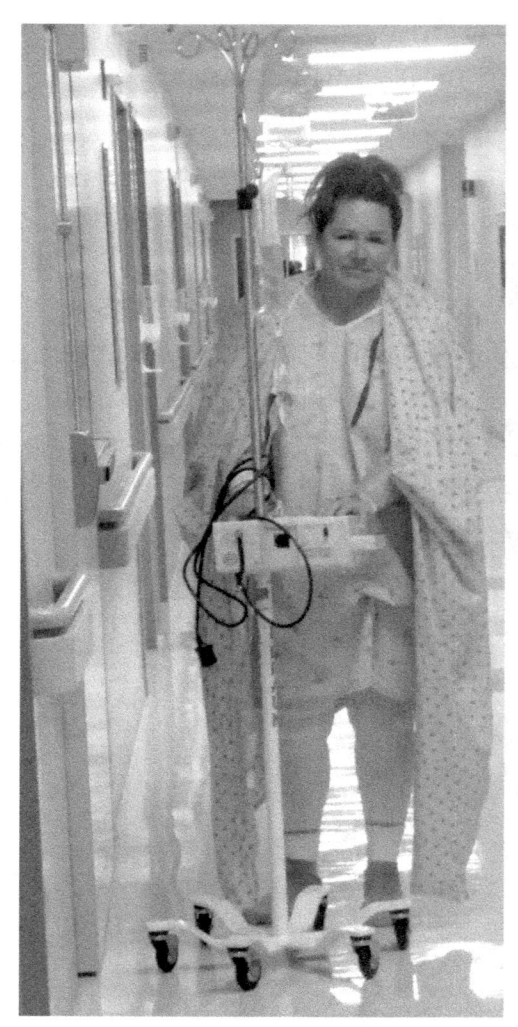

- 7 -

Inches Off at One Week
May 30

Grace measured me the night before surgery. It's one week later and she just took the measurements again.

Neck: .5 inch
Bust: 1.5 inches
Waist: 3 inches
Hips: 3 inches
Thighs: 1.5 inches
Upper arms: .5 inch

So it's not just my imagination. It's real. This is happening. Isn't it funny how you can feel it and see it, your family tells you they can see it, but you need that validation from the scale or the tape measure? I hope one day I don't need to see the numbers to believe I'm healthier. I hope one day I don't even need to question it. I'll just know I'm healthier and get on with living.

- 8 -

Still Doing Great
June 2

It's now 11 days since my surgery and things are going well. I'm functioning on a normal schedule. I'm blessed to be able to work from home many days, so getting to work is easy. But I've run errands to the store, to my mom's, picking up kids from school, football and ballet, and I feel great!

I had some fat-free cream soup last night and it was nice to have something savory. I haven't weighed myself since Monday, and I think I forgot to mention how many pounds off. According to my scale it's 14 pounds since my pre-op appointment! I'll weigh on my surgeon's scale next week.

I've been doing a good amount of walking around my neighborhood, and feeling good doing it. I started some strength training with 5-pound weights. I'm still not hungry. I eat because I need to. I drink because I need to, but I'm not thirsty.

Did you hear that post-op patients? It doesn't matter if you're thirsty or not, DRINK!

So, although I had major surgery last week that will change my life forever, everything else is otherwise back to normal. From my experience so far, if you're thinking about having surgery, if you've already met with a surgeon, or if you're scheduled for surgery...YOU CAN DO THIS! Find your support system through your surgeon's group, your friends and family, and the on-line family of fellow weight loss surgery patients.

- 9 -

My First Party After Surgery
June 5

Yesterday, my family and I attended the baptism of my new Godson, Giovanni. After the ceremony we went to Wood Ranch Restaurant for Kansas City BBQ and there was plenty of it!

I packed a ready-to-drink protein shake and packets of Crystal Light. As soon as we were seated I asked for a glass with ice and a glass of water so I could prepare my drinks. I was already sipping my protein drink when the appetizers started to arrive at the tables; fried onion strings, chicken wings, artichoke dip & chips. Guests were having cocktails and beer. Everyone was having a good time!

And me?

I was okay. My husband kept asking me how I was doing, and my reply was. "I'm okay." Of course the food smelled and looked delicious, and everyone was thoroughly enjoying it, but I was okay. For lunch I ordered Tri-Tip & Mushroom soup. It was so good. I saved the Tri-Tip pieces for my husband, but I slowly chewed and ate the small amounts of carrots and mushrooms in the soup. I continued to drink my protein shake and Crystal Light, and all was well.

KEY FACTORS FOR TODAY'S SUCCESS:
1. **I ordered something and enjoyed it.** My friend told me about her first restaurant experience after surgery and her advice was to order something you can have and enjoy it! Don't sit there feeling sorry for yourself, you can enjoy going out and celebrating!
2. **Be prepared.** I like Crystal Light so having something to drink at the party other than water was important. I took a protein shake with me.
3. **Great benefit of weight loss surgery is I'm still not hungry.** It probably would have been so much harder sitting there, looking at all that food if I was hungry and trying to diet on my own. But not being hungry AND knowing I would be sick if I tried to eat the food is an amazing asset. It's something I couldn't do on my own before surgery.

In the end, Giovanni was baptized, there was a wonderful celebration, and I didn't feel out of place, sad or upset that I couldn't partake in all the delicious food. I enjoyed my soup and drinks, my family and friends, grateful this surgery is working!

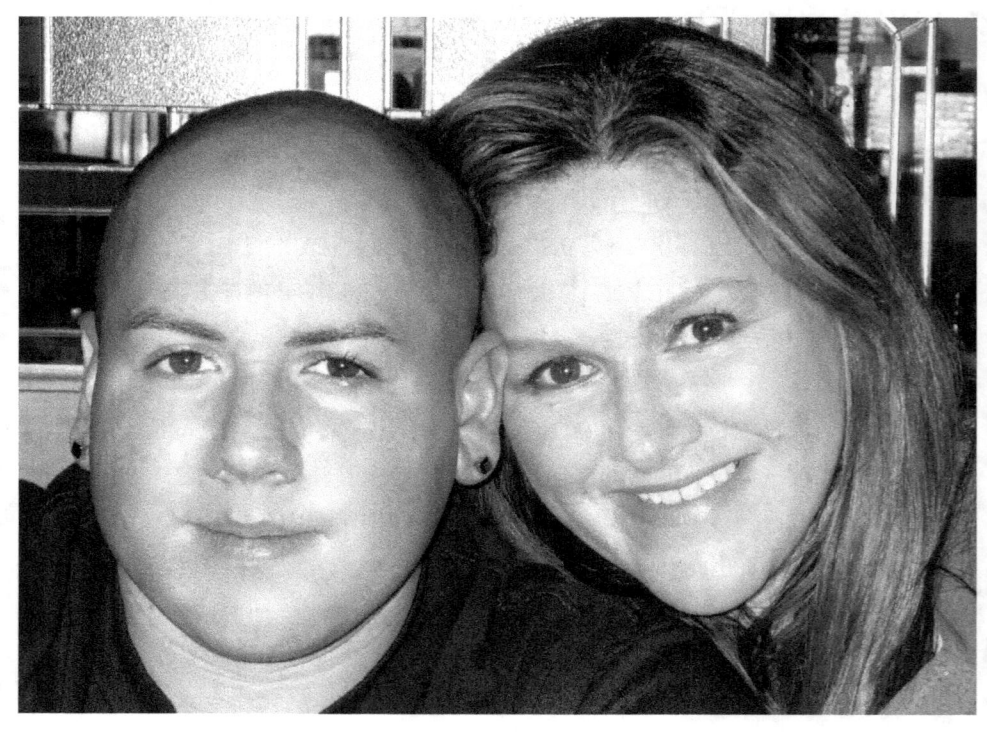

- 10 -

I Haven't Worn These Clothes in 3 Years
June 9

I put on my pants this morning and then came the, "Okay, what top do I wear?" I pulled out my favorite lavender top. I've put it on at least three times in the past year but it never fit. I thought I could wear it with a jacket or sweater, but it never looked right so I always just took it off, feeling horrible. But THIS morning I put it on and it fit with room to spare! I wore it without a jacket and I felt great!

I had tuna last night with a little light-mayo and it was delicious! I'm still enjoying cottage cheese, sugar-free popsicles, Jello and soup.

At work today, my coworker seemed surprised when I told her I was exercising. But I am, and I like it again - 45 minutes daily. The school near my home has steps leading to the front of the school, and in the evening there's a beautiful view. So I go up and down, and I just keep going. Of course my music is on and before you know it,

45 minutes have passed. I continue to use light weights for my arms when I get home. I'm sure the time for exercise was always there, but now I want to do it.

I know the surgery is just a part of the plan for success. It can't do everything. I have a lot to do. And if I don't, I won't get the results I want. So following the nutrition guidelines, exercising, drinking lots of water, taking my vitamins and supplements, and staying POSITIVE...that's my job.

Thank you to my wonderful husband who walks with me in the evenings, and tells me how great I'm doing every day!

- 11 -

And Life Goes On
June 22

Graduations, anniversaries, Father's Day. Where do I begin?

First, things are going well. Any hitches? I've had two occasions when I must have been eating too quickly. I thought I was chewing very well before swallowing, but I was still going too fast. So I had 'tightness'. It wasn't pain, but a feeling that took about 10 minutes to go away. Lying down seemed to help. So I am being more careful with the time I take to eat.

There have been a lot of celebrations lately, and for the most part I've handled them well.

Until Father's Day.

My kids and I decided we'd cook at home. Brunch and then a lasagna dinner. I started food prep on Saturday after shopping at Costco, maybe my first mistake since everything is 10 times as big. I was cooking for four kids, my husband and my mom. And I guess I'm still in the mindset of 'you show your family how much you care for them by making delicious food and plenty of it'. I cooked like I was feeding an army. And here it is Wednesday, and I still have leftovers from breakfast and a full tray of lasagna.

So how do I change my mindset?

Too much food isn't good for me, and it's not good for my family either. I have some changing to do in how my family approaches celebrations.

My birthday is tomorrow and my mom called this morning wanting to know where we're going out to celebrate. She doesn't mean out to the park or the beach, she means out to EAT. It's where our minds automatically turn when planning a celebration. So with the Father's Day food -overload in recent memory, and the remains still in my refrigerator, I need to come up with another solution to FOOD. Getting together to celebrate but not making it about EATING. So, I'm thinking about this.

A change for my birthday this year is I want new cross-trainers. Usually I want a SEPHORA gift card or perfume, never anything exercise-related. But since I'm exercising daily, my old shoes aren't feeling that great. And I'm excited to go shoe shopping!

The pounds are coming off but I still prefer to go by my tape measure and my clothes. It's interesting that some parts of my body lose a little each week consistently. Some don't budge for a couple of weeks and then BOOM - an inch off. Last week I wore jeans a size smaller than when I had surgery. That was pretty cool.

I'm still drinking plenty of water and enjoying new foods. I still love tuna and cottage cheese so they're staples. I made a ratatouille-like dish with onions, garlic, tomatoes, zucchini, yellow squash and ground turkey. Delicious!

All in all, things are going well. There are plenty of things to work on though, with my mind AND my body.

- 12 -

I Swear I Asked Her If It Was Sugar Free
June 24

So yesterday was my birthday, and I got back from work late. Remember I work 85 miles from my house? Anyway, my sweet daughter made me a birthday cake, chocolate with pink flowers. I walked in and there it was with candles aglow! Before I could say anything, Grace said, "Don't worry, Mom. Dad took me to the store and I used sugar-free cake mix and sugar-free frosting."

How sweet of her, right?

Grace served me a small piece. I swallowed the first bite and said, "Wow! Sugar-free cake is really good." I had a second bite, chewed slowly and felt so happy. I waited another five minutes or so, had one more bite, and I was done. Then we all sat down to watch a movie.

Somewhere between 3-5 minutes into the movie, I started to feel weird. It was a mixture of nausea, chills, sweats, and my heart was racing. Then it got worse. I looked at Grace, "You used sugar-free cake mix and frosting right? That's what you said, SUGAR-FREE!" Grace looked at me with the 'uh-oh' face and said, "But I ran out of sugar-free frosting so I had to use regular frosting for the flowers."

I ate full-sugar frosting one month after surgery. Yes, I did.

I walked around, my husband rubbed my shoulders, I went outside, I thought I was going to vomit but I never did. There was nothing else to be done except go to bed. I had to sleep it off.

While I was trying to force myself into sleep, Grace kept saying, "I'm sorry, Mom."

Here's my message. Patients are cautioned to beware of how food is prepared when they eat in restaurants. Cream sauces, marinades, salad dressings…things you forget have a high sugar content. Of course we think patients know what's being prepared in their own homes. So here is my story of warning.

Even at home, sugar shows up.

But here's the thing. I'm glad it happened. Yes, glad. I've always loved sweets. When I was given the option to have a different procedure that didn't really cause dumping, I responded, "NO! I love sweets too much. I know myself too well." It's true. Some people are chips and popcorn people but not me. I'm the ice cream, donut, cookie person. Bring on the dumping!

Okay, well don't just bring it on. I just like knowing that I've experienced it and hopefully that's enough for me to make healthy choices with my food from here on out.

And to check the trash for sugar-free containers when Grace bakes me a cake.

- 13 -

Ten Years in Bariatric Surgery
and I Thought I Knew Everything
June 28

Last week I attended my surgeon's patient education meeting and suport group. I haven't been in months, so I'm glad I did because it was great!

First the Pre-op class:
The room was packed! Patients coming up for surgery and their supportive family and friends. Lots of information is delivered in this 3-hour class, but it's seriously worth the time! As a patient, he refreshed my memory of all the things post-op patients must do to take good care of themselves. He has a great way of connecting with people, making them laugh, making them think. There was lots of interaction and sharing amongst the patients.

I appreciated being able to share a little of my experience with the patients, from the perspective of someone who just had surgery. I was honest, "my back hurt", "you should have someone spend the first night in the hospital with you", "the drain is uncomfortable but you'll get through it". But I was also able to share, "I've been out to eat and I handled it", "I'm not ever hungry. I eat because I need to.", "I can still drink plenty of water, at least 7 bottles a day", "I am VERY happy I did this".

The support group meeting was moderated by our wonderful psychologist, Dr. Irit Gat. She began by giving some topics and the group took it from there. They discussed friends and family members who they feel are jealous of their weight loss, who seem to undermine their success with subtle sabotage. Another topic was worrying before surgery, "Is this going to work for me? Will I ever be able to eat out with my family?" The group was large but everyone respected each other's time when speaking. Again, I was very glad I went. It was a great day!

I got the greatest pair of shoes for my birthday! Reebok REALFLEX. So light and comfortable. Great for walking and a good step-workout.

Exercise is going well and so is eating. Saturday we celebrated my birthday at my mom's, it seemed like the best solution. We made hamburgers, and all the regular picnic-sides. I had a bite of a burger with mustard and tomato, a few bites of a pickle, and a bite of baked beans. Of course this was over time, and it stayed down, no upset stomach. I was fine. My favorites are still cottage cheese, string cheese, yogurt, tuna, ground turkey or chicken, ratatouille, and a vegetable omelet. I drink a lot of water, sometimes with Crystal Light.

You start to get the hang of things after four weeks.

When I was in support group last week, a patient asked a question and I said, "I'm not ever hungry." I heard a man behind me comment, "Honeymoon period," and to some extent I'm sure he's right. I know eventually I will be hungry and I'll have some challenging days. But right now while things are going well, I'm doing all I can to maximize my results.

This weekend my daughter and I went through all the clothes I've been saving, that I love but could no longer fit into.

I have a new wardrobe!

It felt so amazing trying on those clothes and having them just slip on. I remember being in Weight Watchers in the 90s and my leader would say, "Nothing tastes as good as thin feels." I think this statement is very true. But when you're trying to lose weight completely on your own, without the surgery, you know this statement is true and still you eat. Because in the moment the food gives you that pleasure, that release from the stress, that comfort. But while I have it, the feeling of "not hungry," I'm going to embrace it and use it for all its got!

BOTTOM LINE...I chose to have this surgery and I'm choosing to make it work. And it is work, every day. But I have this amazing tool that helps me not crave food or eat a lot, and eat only healthy foods because I'm scared of dumping and cramps, and that's a good thing. I'm finding other ways to cope with things because I have to. I've definitely had experiences, even today, when something caused stress and I found myself thinking about food, wanting to get something to eat. But then I reminded myself, "Mary, you're not even hungry. You're never hungry. So why do you want something to eat?" But this is something that was very hard to do on my own before the surgery. Now I'm forced to think before I eat and that's good.

- 14 -

Here, You Eat It.
July 11

Last week I went to lunch with my friend and coworker. I suggested she get a coffee shake. "Oh no, that's okay, Mary. I don't really want one," she said. But I kept insisting by suggesting she order one to take back to the office. She again politely replied, "No, thank you."

During lunch I told her that my husband said he thought I was feeding the family more than I did before surgery. "The portions are getting bigger and bigger," he told me. A couple days after that, I was driving home from my mom's with my kids and told them, "We should stop and get ice cream cones, and we can get your dad a shake since I can't carry his cone in the car." Now keep in mind, neither of my kids asked for ice cream, nor did my husband ask me to bring him a shake. IT'S ALL ME!

I've been giving my family things I'm not eating anymore. I'm trying to feed them more because I'm eating less!

Where does this come from?

I actually talked with my mom about it. I told her I remembered how much my dad loved food. He was raised in the midwest, heavy food and plenty of it. I remember making my dad a sandwich and knowing that there better be plenty of mayonnaise, cheese and whatever meat I was using. It made him happy. If I served him pie there was plenty of ice cream on top. It's how we showed our love. But my Dad died after a heart attack when he was 60.

Back to lunch with my friend. I was telling her all of this and she said, "Mary, that's what you just did to me!" She's right, that's exactly what I did to her. She's never ordered a shake or iced coffee when we've been out. She doesn't drink with her meals because she had weight loss surgery too! But there I was, insisting she get a treat that I couldn't have. Is it because I really want to see people I care about enjoy things I'm not eating anymore, even though I know those things aren't healthy for them either?

Wow.

My family and I have talked about this now. We've agreed that the whole family will eat more like I've been eating. Protein, vegetables, and small portions of whole grains and fruit. We also agreed that less healthy food like pizza or lasagna aren't off the table, but reserved for once-in-a-while. So this weekend, my daughter said French toast sounded good for breakfast. I used whole grain bread from our local farmer's market, egg beaters and non-stick cooking spray. We also used sugar-free syrup. I warned my family before they sat down to eat that this wouldn't be the French toast they were accustomed to. The result? They loved it.

The lesson for me here is AWARENESS. Being aware of the role food has played in my life, the life of my family, and the role it should play. I still think food is wonderful and to be enjoyed. However, I'm much more aware of all the healthier foods we can enjoy and the rewarding results the healthier food leaves behind.

Bon appetit!

- 15 -

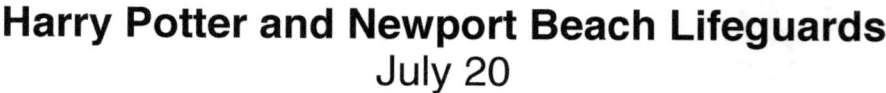

Harry Potter and Newport Beach Lifeguards
July 20

So I'm being asked, "Okay Mary, but how much weight have you lost?" Understandably after weight loss surgery, numbers are a big deal. But as I've written here, SO much more is involved.

But let's talk about it. Grace took my measurements the night before surgery, May 22nd. We took my measurements again this past Monday, July 18th, eight weeks since surgery. Here is the breakdown on how many inches I've reduced in different areas:

Neck: 1.5 inches
Upper arms: 1 inch
Bust: 4 inches
Waist: 8 inches
Hips: 5.5 inches
Thighs: 5 inches

I checked my weight last week. I've lost 35 pounds. I had to go shopping for pants. I thought I had more pants in smaller sizes than I did. I bought two size-14 pants last week. That's down from an 18-20 when I had surgery. It feels great.

When I was shopping I walked past a full length mirror which I'd usually RUN by. So I walked by and then stepped back to look at myself. I stood there and thought, "I look so much better."

That was a huge deal.

I haven't felt that way about myself in years. I kept shopping and realized there were tears in my eyes. I was shopping for smaller sizes. And in the back of my mind, I knew the sizes would only get smaller.

We saw Harry Potter this weekend in the IMAX theater. I can run to the top of the stairs without stopping and when I reach the top, I'm not out of breath. And I can keep talking the whole time.

We went to the beach this weekend, and although I wasn't ready to go out in a swimsuit, I did go out in a sundress. My legs hadn't seen the light of day in years. And aside from my kids getting caught in a wave, requiring help from Newport Beach lifeguards and paramedics, I felt pretty good about my first outing to the beach since surgery.

This is all a process. The food, exercise, vitamins and supplements, clothes, family, friends, the EMOTIONS. It is definitely a daily journey.

My advice so far?
1. Find an exercise you LOVE because you have to do it daily, and you have to want to do it because of what is does for you. Accept that exercise is an important part of your life and will be forever. Integrate it wherever and whenever you can.

2. Get your vitamins and supplements organized. Make sure you're taking everything your surgeon recommends and pay attention to when you take them. Some vitamins and supplements are better absorbed when eaten with different foods. Do your research, ask questions, and plan ahead.

3. After eight weeks I know who genuinely wants to support me and who isn't really interested in my progress…and that's okay. This is MY journey and I can't expect everyone to be on board in a big way. Everybody has their own journeys they're on right now. Their journeys may not be as evident as major weight loss, but everyone is in a process of change and growth.

4. Enjoy the ride! Think about what's going on and don't rush through it. You're learning lessons that will last a lifetime.

5. Be grateful for your family and friends who continue to be there for you, like my husband. The other night, it was about 11 p.m. and I was really tired. But I had taken the first step, putting on my workout clothes and shoes. Then

I sat on the couch. I looked at him and said, "I need your help. I have to work out." He got out my STEPS and asked what movie he could put on that would energize me. So we watched "The Hangover" and time passed so quickly I didn't even know I was going up and down on the steps. Thank you, Honey!

I want to wear a button or shirt that says, "I HAD WEIGHT LOSS SURGERY AND I'M OKAY IF YOU WANT TO ASK ME ABOUT IT!" Okay, maybe that didn't roll off the tongue but you get my point. I want people to know how good they can feel physically and emotionally. I want people to know they can live happier, healthier lives.

Okay I'm off my soap box. If you've already had surgery, you know what I'm talking about. If you're getting ready for surgery you are so lucky! You've been blessed with an amazing opportunity to get your life back and really live it. Congratulations.

- 16 -

I Got in the Water
July 27

We all have our hang-ups and insecurities. When you're extremely overweight (sometimes morbidly obese is hard to type) going swimming in a public place is difficult.

I don't have a pool but I've always enjoyed the water, in private pools with close friends or family. But I know swimming is a nearly-perfect exercise. When I see patients who look really toned, and I ask them what they're doing for exercise, the answer is almost always, "SWIMMING!"

With swimming, weight bearing stress is practically eliminated, the heart enlarges pumping 10-20% more blood per beat, and because of the resistance, 30 minutes in water is like 60 minutes on land. You can't beat that!

Still, with all of this information, I've been hesitant to venture out to our local YMCA. But this morning at 7 am, I dragged Grace out of bed (she actually came willingly) and we went to the Y! It was a matter of following through on each step.

1. Making the decision last night and setting out the towel, swimsuit and flip-flops.
2. Setting the alarm and convincing my daughter to go with me for support.
3. When the alarm went off this morning - making no excuses. "GO!"
4. Walking into the YMCA and getting into the pool.

After this I was home free. I love to swim and I just had to get through this first time in public, and now I'm okay. We swam and did water exercises for over an hour. It was a workout, but relaxing at the same time. I loved it!

So, I can check-off another milestone in my weight loss surgery journey. There are so many! Each day brings another experience to learn from, to grow through. Weight loss surgery is not just about losing the weight, it's so much more. Congratulations to all of you who are making this journey with me. Whether you've just decided to start your journey or you're 10 years out from surgery, it's a blessing, a true blessing.

- 17 -

Reactions
August 10

By reactions, I mean how people react to me, then how I react to them reacting to me. Confusing? Let me explain.

I met my good friend, Lana, for brunch on Saturday. We've known each other for about eight years. She had weight loss surgery about seven years ago and is still doing great! In the days leading up to our brunch date she made jokes like, "Wear a rose in your hair so I know it's you!" When I got out of my car, she shrieked with delight, "Mary! Mary!" We had a great visit and she shared her words of wisdom as a long-term successful weight loss surgery patient.

"Exercise needs to be part of your everyday life. Be cautious about treats. Keep them for really special occasions only. Remember why you had surgery. It was a big deal, so treat it that way. Take care of yourself and keep in mind what you did to get healthy. And don't get caught up in people's reactions to the new you."

I knew the story Lana was about to tell me. Soon after surgery, her sister stopped talking to her. It was hard for Lana because she didn't understand why. It was almost a year before her sister called her and said, "I've been avoiding you and I'm sorry. For the last 20 years I've been the thin sister. You had the better job, the close group of friends, and being thin was my thing. I'm sorry I didn't return your calls. I'm sorry I wasn't there for you."

Last week I went walking early in the morning and passed my neighbor watering his front yard. We said our customary, "Good morning," and then he said, "hey, looking good!" That felt wonderful and weird at the same time. I thought about it more while I was walking. My neighbors see me nearly every day. They knew how big I had gotten, so of course they're likely to notice if I've dropped a few clothing sizes over the last couple of months. And I don't think it's only my size they're noticing. I already look healthier and happier than I did before surgery.

Yesterday I ran into a close family member. She hasn't seen me in about a month. We were in a parking lot, and when I came out from between two cars and she saw all of me she remarked, "Wow," but in a kind of "Oh," kind of way. This family member has always been slim, so this is an interesting new dynamic.

It's another part of the weight loss surgery journey.

Along with eating healthy, consuming enough protein,

drinking plenty of water, taking vitamins, and exercising daily, there are the social, mental, and emotional factors. They're very real and you can't ignore them.

Again, I emphasize that every step in this journey is an opportunity for growth. Learning how good I can feel after an hour-long swim, how it doesn't even feel like exercise, and wanting to do it again tomorrow. Learning that I can enjoy a party without trying everything on the buffet table and still have a good time. Understanding that bottom line, this is my body, my life, and my health. Understanding that every decision I make affects me.

I'm doing my best to make good choices. I've been given a second chance to have a healthy life, and God willing I'll make the most of it.

I'm going to a family reunion this weekend. This is the first time in a LONG time that I haven't gone through the self-induced stress of dieting before an event.

"The party is four weeks away and I can lose 15 pounds, no problem!"
"It's two weeks away, I can still lose 10 pounds if I eat only one meal a day."
"It's not too late, one week away and I can lose 7 pounds if I follow the Scarsdale diet,"

And then I would lose nothing and be depressed about it. I'm done with that now.

- 18 -

Spread the News
September 12

I've worked in this field for more than ten years and back when I started, bariatric surgery teams had to do a lot of education. Information about the surgeries wasn't as abundant as it is now. People knew something about it, especially after Carnie Wilson became the poster-child with live images of her gastric bypass surgery in 1999. But there was still so much to teach people.

What's interesting is how much is still misunderstood about weight loss surgery a decade later. Sadly, much of the general public is not informed. Even worse is that some health professionals can be misinformed. This becomes a problem when they speak as if they really know what they're talking about because it discourages those who could really benefit from the surgery.

At a recent gathering, I shared my weight loss surgery experience with a small group of friends and acquaintances, including a registered nurse with more than 25 years on the job. The group had a lot of questions:

"But all you can eat is liquids, right?"
"It's hard on the family, isn't it?"
"I heard you're out of work for at least six weeks because they cut you down the middle?"

I answered all their questions and then my 15-year old son, Adrian, answered their question about the surgery's effect on the family. "No, it's not bad. I'm happy for my mom. And we just eat better now too."

The nurse remarked that she's had two patients in her clinic suffering terribly from dumping caused by their weight loss surgery, "It's a defect of the surgery," she said authoritatively. She went on to describe their symptoms of nausea, stomach cramps, vomiting, and hot flashes.

I jumped in. "If they're experiencing those symptoms, it does sound like dumping. But that also means they're causing their own symptoms by the choices they're making." I explained to the group what dumping is and what causes it. It seemed to make sense to them, even the nurse. I went on to say that I had experienced dumping about a month after surgery and was happy I did!

"I have this amazing internal tool that alerts me in a BIG way when I'm eating what I shouldn't, and I need that!"

This past weekend, a woman I see weekly at my aunt's assisted living center, commented about my weight loss.

"I had weight loss surgery," I told her. I don't hide how I'm losing weight. I want people to know about weight loss surgery and how their lives can be transformed. It turns out she had pursued the surgery a few years ago but couldn't afford the co-insurance payment for the hospital. Since then, her pre-diabetes has evolved into diabetes type 2 and she's miserable. I encouraged her to check back into it and she responded, "Yes, I should. But I'm nearing the age when I won't be eligible anymore." I told her there is no official age limit, that my surgeon just operated on a 74-year old woman two months ago. She was shocked to hear that. She'd heard that 60 was the cut-off age.

Years ago, weight loss surgery patients didn't always share the details about how they lost 100 pounds or more. I believe more patients are speaking openly about it now and sharing why they chose to have it, and I love this! Because we all know that without weight loss surgery it was impossible to reduce our weight and keep it off. And I am saddened when people don't pursue it because of misinformation. I believe that we, as weight loss surgery patients, have received an extraordinary gift. And by accepting this gift, we should share the news with those who need to hear it as much as we did.

- 19 -

My Brain Can't Keep Up With My Body
September 19

I've attended multiple bariatric surgery workshops and conferences, including courses on the Psychological Aspects of Weight Loss Surgery at the annual American Society for Metabolic and Bariatric Surgery meetings. And yet, all of this doesn't exclude me from having the same experiences as other patients.

When does your brain finally catch up with what's happening to your body? I'm running out of clothes, and while that sounds like an amazing problem to have and I know it is, it's still something to deal with. So off to the store I go.

I know my large shirts are a little big but I can't bring myself to think I'd fit into a medium. Prior to surgery, I wouldn't even try the clothes on. I'd just guess if I could fit into the item and take it home to try on. If the clothes didn't fit at home, I'd take them back. Now I'm trying the clothes on in the store. I took medium and large into the dressing room. The medium top fit perfectly. Huh? When I look at the top on the hanger, when I hold it up, I cannot accept that there is any way this top will fit me. It's not possible. IT'S NOT POSSIBLE! But you know what's even more shocking? I need smaller jeans again.

If you're reading this and you're in the pre-op phase, you may think I'm bragging or rubbing your face in it. I would have thought exactly the same thing, so I get it. But these are real feelings you need to be ready for. It takes time to process all the changes you go through physically, mentally, and emotionally.

The best thing? This surgery works!

Of course you have to continue to make it work for you. Your protein, vitamins and supplements, water, exercise, plenty of sleep, determination and patience!

Best of health to you all.

- 20 -

You Never Know How Soon You'll Need This
September 26

L ast week my surgeon taught his pre-op education class to about 40 eager patients. The exciting changes that are coming are amazing and these patients have every right to be thrilled. But I still think many patients skip over the importance of developing coping skills for those times when we used to use food for comfort and distraction.

The surgery, no matter which type, does its job very well. But as my surgeon emphasizes again and again,"The surgery is a tool. It doesn't do the whole job." And it's true, it doesn't.

I've said before that now I have this amazing tool which allows me to control my eating. I've said to embrace this new tool, seize it and make it your own. But if you count only on the surgical intervention to lose and control your weight and disregard lifestyle management, you're robbing yourself of the full impact of weight loss surgery.

Right now my family and I are going through a stressful time. A really difficult, hard time. Prior to surgery, food would have been my go to solution to reduce stress. And at 4-months post-op, there are things I could probably eat to deal with the stress. Not much, but I could snack throughout the day. But I'm not. I won't say I'm handling this stressful time perfectly, but better than I would have before surgery.

Working in this field and teaching patients how to mentally prepare for how they'll deal with stress after surgery, I gave it strong consideration myself. I embraced exercise early on. It was challenging in the beginning, but very soon I began to love it again. And now, exercise is my life saver. I'm actually doing what they say to do when you're stressed. I go for a walk or a hike, and before surgery that was so much easier said than done. Without exercise, this stress I'm going through could have been unmanageable. I vary my exercise with walking, steps at the school, swimming, weights, Pilates, and brace yourself...jogging. Yes, jogging. Okay, it was me who needed to brace myself just to tell you that.

The other day I was in a rush to pick-up my son from his haircut and then get back to pick up my daughter from an appointment. I parked the car and ran across the street into the salon, then back across the street to the car. I got into the car and said to my son, "Oh my goodness, I can run. I'm not even out of breath!" So I started jogging a little that evening. At first I actually felt silly. I still have it in my head that I must look ridiculous jogging. But I don't. Nobody's looking at me weird. I'm just a woman jogging down the street.

Love and support from your family during stressful times is so important, and children give us the purest form of love and support.

I was in the car with my son a few days ago, sitting in traffic. For some reason my knees caught my attention, and as I rubbed them I said, "Wow, I have knees." Adrian got irritated and replied, "Mom! Stop saying stuff like that!" I told him I didn't understand why he was getting so upset about me pointing out that I could finally see my knee-caps. He explained,"Mom, I know you're happy about losing weight and I'm happy for you. But when you say stuff like that it's like you're saying that something was wrong with you before. You're the same mom to me. You take care of me, you love me, and you're always there for me." Adrian has no idea, even though I tried to tell him, how much that meant to me, particularly because of what just happened to our family.

If you're in the pre-op stage, you're going for tests, meeting with the dietitian, psychologist, and just trying to do everything you can to be ready for the big day. It's easy to get caught up in the physical stuff and think that the mental stuff will just work itself out after surgery. But like everything important in life, you must put the work into it and prepare. Stress management, exercise, support, loving friends and family. Put just as much effort into these areas, please. You never know how soon after surgery you'll need them. I didn't. But yet, here I am.

- 21 -

I'm Trying Not to Miss a Thing
October 10

It's been four and a half months since surgery, and for the most part I feel like I've got a handle on it. But life keeps going, and sometimes it seems to be going faster than it did before. That's probably because as your weight reduces your energy increases. And with increased energy we schedule more things into our days. However, with a commitment to healthier eating and daily exercise comes more planning, preparation and action. And this takes more time. But being able to be more active is such a blessing. And this isn't just a reference to exercise.

Recently, I visited Coffee Bean & Tea Leaf to buy my aunt's favorite tea. The place was packed. The tea display was in a corner behind groups of people huddled around tables, and there wasn't much room for me to get through. But here's where the new confidence kicks in. I see a spot between two tables and I know I can fit through there. I make my way over confidently, pass through the chairs and get the tea! If you're reading this and you've never been severely overweight, you won't understand what an accomplishment this is. To not have your weight be an obstacle to something as simple as buying a tin of tea! These moments come around more often and I try not to miss them. I pay attention so I can recognize and appreciate them.

I'm doing my labs this week and I hope they come out okay. I really do my best to get everything in. My multi-vitamin, calcium, iron, B12, Biotin, Fish and Flax Oil. And remember, these are what I need. Yours may be different so check with your surgeon. But I do miss one or two here and there, so I'm glad I'm getting my labs done. I need to know if I'm meeting my body's needs.

I'm excited about a new project I'm working on. I'm getting a group of my weight loss surgery friends together to create a kind of mentor team. I knew it before but not to the extent I do now, realizing after having surgery myself how important it is to hear about the experiences, insights, and advice from patients who have gone before you. My goal is to gather women and men of all ages, procedure types and all stages of the weight loss surgery journey. My intention is to offer real-world experience to other patients, whether they're just beginning to consider surgery, or are only a few months behind us in their post-op journeys. REAL experience matters. My 10+ years working in the field still doesn't compare to my 5 months as a patient. It's like anything else. When you've walked in the shoes, you understand the journey.

I remain extremely grateful that I was able to have this surgery and that everything has been going well with it. Again, you need to do the work, but the benefits are unbelievable. Physical, social, spiritual, mental, and emotional. No matter where you are in your journey, embrace your new strength, follow your surgeon's instructions, and do everything within your power to get the maximum results possible. You deserve it!

- 22 -

Waiting for the Other Shoe to Drop
October 20

The decision to have weight loss surgery is a big one, right? And even though we knew all the tremendous statistics before we had surgery, like how effective it is long-term, we still had our doubts. I know I did.

Everything is going so well, you almost wonder when the other shoe will drop. But then you calm down and begin to consider everything rationally. The long-term studies demonstrate that patients who commit to bariatric nutrition, vitamins, daily exercise, and monitoring their lifestyles consistently, have the greatest success with long-term weight control. So instead of panicking, I need to be accountable.

The reasons I decided to have surgery may be similar to yours.

My health. Resolve my diabetes, improve my liver function, decrease symptoms of my Rheumatoid Arthritis, eliminate and decrease my need for multiple medications for my other conditions.

My quality of life. To not wake up every morning focused on my weight, feeling guilty about it, depressed about it, angry about it, sad about it. To wake up and live without the burden of being obese. Seeing it, feeling it, thinking about it almost constantly. To feel better physically, mentally and emotionally. To be able to live without limitations.

So how's it going at almost 5-months post-op?

It's going well. But what about accountability? Well, first I am accountable to myself. I remind myself about how long I struggled with obesity, and how it complicated my life. I acknowledge the 'miracle' of weight loss surgery, and how if you follow all the guidelines, what the studies say is true. It works. At the end of each day I recall where I was successful and where I need to pay more attention to my surgeon's guidelines. Then I make adjustments for the next day. And there are adjustments EVERY DAY. It's okay though. The important thing is I'm aware.

I'm accountable to my family and close friends, and I guess even to people I barely know because I'm open and honest about how I've reduced my weight. Somehow, talking about it openly helps me stay accountable. I believe in the surgery and want other people who need it to know there's hope for them too. I tell my family and close friends if I'm struggling, forgetting to take my vitamins, or not getting in enough protein. Usually, just the process of stating my shortcomings out loud makes me more aware and puts me back in check. Then I decide what to do differently the next day. And sometimes their observations and suggestions are just what I need to get back on track.

I do have a slight advantage in knowing so many post-op patients with many becoming good friends. I learn from their experiences as they're further along than I am, between 3-7 years since surgery. They tell me what their struggles have been and how they've overcome them. They tell me what to watch out for and why.

The support of my weight loss surgery friends is invaluable. You may find like me, that connecting with other patients becomes a huge factor in your journey. Consider striking up a conversation with your fellow patients when you visit your surgeon's office. Attend your local bariatric surgery support group and exchange e-mail addresses or phone numbers. Join a bariatric surgery support group on Facebook, or post a message on your surgeon's Facebook page to connect with your fellow patients.

Bottom line, reach out.

You're not in this alone and it's too important and too challenging to go it alone. Ask for help, ask for support. We deserve ALL this surgery has to offer. Embrace it all and make it yours!

One more thing, some of you have asked and I guess it has been a while so here's the update!

Inches off as of of October 16, 2011

Neck: 2 inches
Arms: 2.5 inches
Bust: 9 inches
Waist: 13 inches
Hips: 10 inches
Thighs: 7 inches

I know this is amazing, and I'm so grateful for these physical changes. But I want to tell you, and I wish I had the words to do it justice, that what I have gained in awareness and understanding about myself is equal to, if not greater than what I've lost in weight.

I didn't expect this. Of course I didn't know the dramatic life-events that were heading my way only 3 months after surgery either. But I know for sure, I would be in a much more difficult place in my life if I hadn't had my surgery when I did.

I guess that's the lesson. You don't know when those life-changing events are going to show up. So it's on us to be prepared as much as we can. Good health, happy spirit, loving and supportive friends and family.

- 23 -

Here's the Proof
October 25

I had labs in late June, about 5 weeks after surgery, so things weren't that dramatically different. But now, WOW! At just about 5 months after surgery the improvements are beyond amazing.

LIVER: With obesity and all the medications I'd taken for more than six years for my conditions, my liver results were already poor. In fact, my surgeon did a liver biopsy when I had my surgery and a little piece of my liver was sent to pathology. The results showed Steatohepatitis with early fibrosis, Non-alcoholic Fatty Liver Disease. This condition is caused by obesity, diabetes, high cholesterol, and metabolic syndrome.

The healthy range for this lab result is: 14-54
My result in March, 2011: 135
My result in October, 2011: 25

LIPID PANEL:

Cholesterol:	3/2011: 197	10/2011: 154
LDL:	3/2011: 107	10/2011: 83
Triglyceride:	3/2011: 98	10/2011: 76
HD Lipoprotein:	3/2011: 3.2	10/2011: 2.8

HEMOGLOBIN A1C: Diabetes

3/2011: 7.5

6/2011: 7.3

10/2011: 6.3

Now this one I was concerned about, because the range is 4.8-5.9. But my surgeon said this is great news because it's gradually coming down.

By the way, have I told you about the day I found out I had diabetes?

In May, 2010, I was at the office and my coworker said, "There's a Dr. Tracy on the phone for you." Okay, everybody knows when the doctor herself is calling you instead of an assistant, it's not good. I got on the phone with my Rheumatologist and she said, "Mary, your lab results came back. It shows your blood glucose is 411. If this is accurate, you should be in a coma right now." She told me I needed to get to a lab immediately and see if the result was accurate or not. I did get to the lab. They ran the test STAT.

My blood glucose was 420.

My eyesight had been blurry, and I'd been feeling like I had the flu. Just that weekend, my husband was barbecuing with the kids and I couldn't even bring myself to get out of bed. This had been my biggest fear, one that I was sure was coming ever since I had gestational diabetes with my kids...I finally had Type 2 Diabetes.

Okay, back to now. So the scale says I'm healthier, the tape measure says I'm healthier, my clothing size says I'm healthier, and now the proof is in the blood, just in case there was any doubt. I AM HEALTHIER!

The body is so brilliantly resilient. During times of our lives when we'd put a lot of effort into eating right and exercising, we'd see the results very quickly. But those efforts weren't sustainable for us. With weight loss surgery, our results ARE SUSTAINABLE. And to see the proof in black and white when I'm looking at my lab results, it's even greater validation that I made the right decision to have surgery and make my life better in every way.

There are some improvements I need to make though. My iron is low so I need to be more diligent about making sure I get in the right amount of supplements and incorporate more iron-rich foods into my meals.

Red meat
Egg yolks
Dark, leafy greens
Turkey
Beans, lentils, chick peas and soybeans

And for good absorption I need to eat them with foods high in Vitamin C:

Cauliflower & Broccoli
Citrus fruits
Green and red bell peppers
Honeydew
Kiwi
Papaya
Strawberries
Tomatoes

Taking care of yourself after surgery is a challenge. For most of us, we didn't dedicate much time to taking care of our health before surgery so this is a BIG lifestyle change. But we made the commitment to do it when we signed our surgical consent. We committed to lifelong health. And nothing great comes easily. This takes daily planned effort. But it is so worth it.

Take advantage of all your surgery has to offer. Make the benefits your own. Enjoy your triumphs each day, you deserve this.

- 24 -

Cross-Addiction
November 10

I've talked about awareness before, in mid-July when it was brought to my attention that instead of giving myself sweet treats, I was pushing my family and friends to eat them since I couldn't.

Experts say food can become a drug that comforts, soothes and numbs the pain, anger, fear, sadness, loneliness, or depression. Everyone has feelings like these, but not everyone uses food. Some use alcohol, recreational drugs, prescriptions drugs, shopping, gambling, sex and even exercise. And of course there are many who've learned to use more productive methods to work through their feelings and stress. The lessons they've learned are the lessons we as weight loss surgery patients need to make sure we master.

I never considered myself a food addict, using food to help myself cope with stress, anger, sadness or fear. But since

I'm out in the open now, I totally did. And over the past 10 years, rarely have I heard weight loss surgery patients openly share that they used food as their coping strategy. I know there are other contributing factors to obesity, but overeating and eating unhealthy food is certainly part of it. So now we've had this surgery, we're taking supplements, exercising, practicing lifestyle management skills, and it's not easy.

I visited an on-line weight loss surgery support group recently to see what post-op patients are talking about. Cross-addiction was receiving as much attention as exercise. I read a post from a woman who developed cross-addiction to alcohol. She had her first drink of champagne at a graduation dinner about three months after surgery and loved how it made her feel. She said within two weeks she was finishing a bottle of wine in three days, then two days, then one day. Finally, her husband found some empty bottles and confronted her. She said she was embarrassed but grateful. The woman described this whole ordeal happening within only two months, "It all happened so quickly." She said she'd never been a drinker but realized about a month into the drinking that she was finding the same comfort in alcohol as she had found before surgery with food. "I liked having a secret comfort that helped me get through the day, just like food had done for me for years and years," she wrote.

I'm happy this woman has a loving husband who confronted her and helped her get into therapy so she could deal with her drinking and what was causing it. She says she's in the process of finding out why she's scared, angry, and sad, and what she can do to overcome these feelings so she's more secure with herself.

This story hit home for me.

My beautiful friend, Lori, had weight loss surgery and was following all the guidelines until she started drinking about six months after surgery. I didn't know she was drinking until she finally told me about a year later. It turns out Lori had been drinking at home every night. I tried to talk with her about it but she was embarrassed, then defensive. She didn't want help from anyone, including her surgeon or his team. Lori's story gets worse. Over the next two years she began using drugs and left her family. There were periods of time when no one knew where she was living, and those who ran into her said she was completely emaciated. Five years after surgery, legal issues became part of her situation and she had no communication with her family or friends. Then, I received the call I knew would eventually come. Loving, kind, sweet Lori, had died at the age of 35. She was a beautiful woman, inside and out, and I miss her.

This is a very personal story for me to share, and although it happened more than four years ago, I haven't told many patients or colleagues about it. But now, as a post-op patient myself, I see the need to emphasize the importance of life and stress management which definitely includes coping skills. We're told so often before weight loss surgery that it doesn't magically make all your troubles go away. The financial, relationship, and employment problems will still be there. The goal is that with improved or resolved medical conditions and with your body at a healthy weight,

weight loss surgery patients are better equipped to handle life's problems.

Experts recommend the following, no matter what your cross-addiction may be.

1. Once you recognize that feeling shame about cross-addiction is normal, don't isolate yourself. Reach out to a trusted friend, family member or fellow weight loss surgery patient. Contact your surgeon, psychologist, or physician. They want to help you.

2. Start a journal, an emotional diary that includes listing situations that trigger stress, anger, sadness, loneliness, fear, shame or depression. Are these situations similar to when you used food to cope, but now you're using something else? Make notes about this and share it with a professional.

3. Either attend your local support group in person, or find an on-line support group that meets your needs.

4. Talk with your trusted family and friends who love you and have shown they care about your well-being. They want to help you be successful and overcome the cross-addiction obstacle. Let them help you.

Please, let people help you.

Continue to be aware and alert each day. Stay healthy, from the inside out.

- 25 -

Holidays and Food Fog
November 24

Mission accomplished. I just made it through the first major eating holiday since surgery.

Another step in the journey.

Thanksgiving seems to be all about the food. Before 9 am, I received five text messages from friends and family who were extending their good wishes with, "Happy Thanksgiving and enjoy feeding your pie hole!" and "Eat all day, don't worry about it until tomorrow!" Yes, it's all about the food. So after weight loss surgery it's not that you can't be excited about food too, it just becomes excitement of a different kind.

It was still fun to plan the menu with Grace.

While I was at work she made the mashed potatoes and appetizers, while other family members were pitching in with different dishes.

Thanksgiving morning I made a holiday breakfast and enjoyed everything the family was eating, but only a few bites because the food was more rich than usual. I made two more dishes for Thanksgiving dinner before heading to my sister's and all was well.

At dinner, I asked Grace to put a tablespoon of everything on my plate. Now a tablespoon of each dish sure doesn't seem like much, and there were some jokes at the table about "Poor Mary," but when you consider all the dishes at a Thanksgiving dinner, my daughter passed back a plate that was FULL! So I dug in like everybody else.

Wow, that was fast.

I filled up quickly because I still observe the protein first rule which meant turkey first. I had a little more as the family sat at the table talking, but by the end of dinner half the food was still on my plate. I had some pumpkin pie with homemade whipped cream and it was delicious. I helped put all the leftovers away and wasn't tempted to snack because I was still full. All in all, I made it through the biggest eating day of the year and I never felt left out just because I wasn't pigging out.

I enjoyed my whole family. My 7-year old nephew's centerpiece, my 89-year old mother teaching him how to play Chinese checkers, my 92-year old aunt eating almost as much as my 15-year old son, my sister telling stories about the funnier side of police work, and then watching everybody fall asleep around the house within 30 minutes of finishing dinner. This left my mother and me, the only ones who didn't pig out, to finish the clean-up. It was all good.

So it's the next day and there's a month of eating opportunities ahead.

Christmas baking, parties, get-togethers, Starbuck's red-cups, and all the rest. And here's what I've been figuring out since surgery and it's becoming more clear with every event, holiday and even every stressful situation.

Wait, I'm getting teary-eyed as I try to come up with the right words...it's not about the food. The event or celebration still happens, even without the food.

Yesterday, my sister's oven went on the fritz after the turkey came out and biscuits went in. It took almost 60 minutes for the biscuits to bake and we were done with dinner by the time they came out. But it was okay. Yes, I realize it wasn't the whole dinner, but it reminded me that we were okay with what we had on the table. I'm becoming more and more okay with what I have in my life, that doesn't revolve around food. Celebrating with less food is completely doable. Looking for and being grateful for the joys of a celebration that have nothing to do with food, is possible. Very possible.

It's like coming out of a food fog.

There's been so much more to holidays and celebrations

other than the food. And stress? There's so many other things we can do besides eat. After surgery, if we allow it, we can open ourselves up to experience so much more without so much food. Through painful experiences we can learn and grow instead of numbing our feelings with food. Through joyful experiences we can embrace the time with our family and friends and make beautiful memories.

During the next 30 days or so, you'll have more opportunities to eat more and richer food than at any other time of year. Remind yourself every morning why you chose to have surgery and why you're grateful that you did. Then make a daily commitment to consume your protein, water, supplements, and to exercise. At the end of each day, your sense of accomplishment will empower you to wake up the next morning and continue to take excellent care of yourself, again.

I wish you fortitude, determination and happiness!

- 26 -

Evolution
December 19

Try to remember the first time you thought about wanting to lose weight. I don't even mean when you first considered weight loss surgery, but the first time you wanted to lose ten pounds. What about the 20th time or the 100th time?

There've been so many different reasons we wanted to lose weight. And when we finally decided to have weight loss surgery we can remember the deciding factors:

"I don't want my knees to hurt anymore,"
"I want more confidence,"
"I want to be off medication,"
"I want to be able to play with my kids or grandkids,"
"I want to shop in regular clothing stores,"
"I just want to feel better."

But now 6 months out, 1, 2 or 5 years out, the motivation

for continuing to lose weight or maintain weight loss has changed, right?

For me, I wanted to reverse and resolve my diabetes. I wanted so badly for my diabetes to be gone that I remember telling my surgeon, "If I could have this surgery and the only thing I'd get from it is my diabetes going away and nothing else, I would still do it." At that time, I was injecting insulin, was on multiple medications, testing my blood, and I hated it.

Now my diabetes is resolved.

I was diagnosed with Rheumatoid Arthritis in 2004. I took many different medications which led to liver problems. Eventually, I had to take injections to prevent further damage. Now, my RA symptoms are almost non-existent. The condition is there, but I'm managing without medication.

So, now that these medical conditions and my others are resolved or in remission and asymptomatic, what's my motivation to continue to lose weight or to maintain my weight loss?

First, if I regain my weight, my diabetes WILL come back. My RA can worsen and my symptoms can come back with a vengeance.

Second, I'm enjoying being a smaller size. Yes, this means it's more fun to shop, but more than that - it's how I exist. My energy level, removal of limitations of what I can do, what I can accomplish, these are things I never thought possible when I was morbidly obese. When I go places I'm not thinking about how other people are perceiving me and my obesity. I love waking up every morning thinking about the blessings of my day ahead and not waking up already disgusted by my weight, what I did wrong the day before, and how I'm a failure.

But as with all great things, and going from morbid obesity to a normal weight is certainly great, there is work involved.

I'm a visual learner. I need to have visual reminders of why I must eat healthy, exercise, take my vitamins and supplements, and get my labs done. One reminder is pictures of me in my home.

Does that sound vain?

If you've been morbidly obese you already know what I mean. There were NO pictures of me in my home, except those taken before I became morbidly obese. So there weren't any pictures of me with my kids at their current ages, or with my granddaughter, or with friends, or at special events. And now there are. It's actually strange to see, but it's important in reminding me why I must do things to stay on track with my weight loss surgery.

Next, there's a Gratitude Wall in my kitchen. My kids and I list the things we're grateful for each day, from the simple to the amazing. And I finally started a journal. From time to time in my life, I've recorded certain events, struggles and accomplishments, but not on a regular basis. Now I am and I love it. It's a reminder of how far I've come, what my triggers are for wanting to eat, what I did to overcome an unhealthy impulse, and how I celebrated my accomplishments. I can look back and see that on the days I had a great workout, ate really healthy and took my vitamins, it directly correlated to what I achieved in my day. But days when I wasn't on track, I didn't get as much done. It's been an interesting journey to observe on paper for sure!

I want to remain free of diabetes and the debilitating effects of Rheumatoid Arthritis (there were times when I couldn't even dress myself or drive to work), and my other conditions.

I want to continue to live a life free of voices in my head telling me that people are judging me, and that I'm not good enough, and that I'm a failure because of my obesity.

I want to live to my fullest potential and be an example for my children and grandchildren.

Well, this takes effort, dedication and perseverance. Am I willing to continue to do the daily work?

Excuse me, I need to grab a water bottle and hit the local Greenway Trail for a walk with my daughter.

Best of life and best of health!

- 27 -

The Journey or the Destination
January 11

Oprah was asked which is more important, the journey or the destination. She immediately responded, "The journey, absolutely."

I know it's true. The Journey is what teaches us, it's how we grow and learn important lessons so we can make the most of ourselves and our lives. But **The Journey** is hard.

Seriously hard.
Difficult.
Challenging.
Frustrating.
Scary.
It's all of these things.

But more than this, The Journey is wonderful, if we really take the time to see it for what it is and appreciate it.
And with weight loss surgery there is no final destination,

not even when you reach your goal weight. It takes continual effort to maintain your weight, maintain your vitamin and mineral levels, to stay healthy.

It's the New Year and I, like you, have settled into life after the holidays. I'm reassessing where I am in my weight loss surgery journey and I'm in the process of making adjustments. There is ALWAYS room for improvement and sometimes not just room for it, but an absolute necessity for it.

Here are some of my **Let's Do Better With This** areas.

Vitamins and Supplements:
I had my labs again and was grateful to see that in most areas I'm doing well. But my iron is still low. It was low the last time I had my labs. And although I vowed to improve it, it's still low. It's not enough to just take 2 iron supplements daily. I need to know how many milligrams I'm taking and what foods I'm consuming near the time I take them so the iron is absorbed properly. I need to buy iron-rich foods and once they're home...I need to actually prepare and eat them. Many times I've had the bag of baby spinach in the refrigerator, I only used for one meal, and then I let it go bad. This thing takes planning and follow-through.

Making Myself a Priority:
In my early 20s, I was a divorced mom with two young boys. I was just beginning my self-improvement education and read that single moms should make themselves a priority. I remember telling my own mom about this. She grew up during the Great Depression, eating only what was

grown in her backyard and going without shoes during the summer because they could only afford one new pair at the beginning of the school year. "Mom, I have to make myself a priority. My needs are important. If I take care of myself my kids will be happier." This message didn't resonate with my mom, and it must not have resonated with me either. I practiced for a few years but with a new husband and three more kids, I was on the back burner again.

What did that get me?
Rheumatoid arthritis, Fibromyalgia, Hashimoto's, liver disease, insulin-dependent diabetes, and morbid obesity. Now I'm in remission from all of them. But having weight loss surgery was only the beginning. To maintain and even continue to improve my health, I choose to make myself a priority. Am I always great at it? No. But I'm practicing every day.

How about you?
On the list of things you have to do today, are you in the top 5?

And I don't mean…

"Sure, I plan on exercising at some point," or "If everything else gets done I might make a healthy dinner."

I'm asking if you have specific things listed as priorities to take care of yourself. What are your boundaries around those priorities? Have you practiced what you'll do or say if your boundaries are challenged?

Boundary challenge #1:
Tuesday, 6 am – planning my day.
Me: "I'll work out tonight between 6-8 pm while my daughter is at dance class."

Tuesday, 5:30 pm – getting dressed for my workout, friend calls.

Friend: "Hey, we haven't see each other in a while and I'll be near your house tonight around 6:30. Let's have coffee!"

Me: "I'd love to, but I've already made a commitment to myself to work out tonight during that time. But I'm available after 8 pm if that'll work for you. If not, let's plan a date for next week."

To some, and maybe even to you, it may sound selfish to put your workout before coffee with a good friend. But turn that around. How does it feel to put yourself last? To blow off your commitment to yourself? My guess...that doesn't feel very good.

Boundary challenge #2:
Saturday, 7:30 am – planning my day.
Me: "I've got vegetables in the refrigerator and I really need to use them. I'll make grilled chicken and roasted vegetables for dinner tonight."

Saturday, 4:00 pm – getting ready to make dinner, kids enter the kitchen.

Kids: "Mom, we don't want chicken and vegetables. Come

on, let's go out for pizza and then get ice cream!"

Me: "I love pizza and ice cream too. But tonight we're having grilled chicken and roasted vegetables. But, we can go for frozen yogurt after dinner."

And of course there CAN be compromise. You don't live in a bubble, so there will be times when you choose to be flexible. But make sure it feels good to you.

Boundary challenge #3:
Sunday, 3 pm – enjoying a family celebration.

Me: "Oh my gosh they're serving Aunt Jenny's homemade lasagna! I haven't had that in forever! I'm sure if I eat slowly maybe I can have two servings throughout the day if I pace myself."

Sunday, 3:15 pm – eating first serving of lasagna.

Me: "This is delicious, but who am I kidding? I'll be lucky if I can finish half of this. I've enjoyed it. It brought back some wonderful childhood memories, and I'm done."

Setting boundaries with friends and family takes practice but eventually most people will learn to respect your choices. The more chalenging work can be setting boundaries with yourself.

Commitment to Exercise:
My exercise routine is allowing me to maintain a size I had not imagined possible just a year ago. But I'm in

my mid 40s and even if I hadn't had weight loss surgery, maintaining a healthy weight would still be a challenge. My current exercise routine was great 3 months ago, but my body has adjusted. I've added a few things to make it more challenging but I'm still counting on the same standards that I'm comfortable with. It's a a little scary to completely change my workout. I'm comfortable doing my workouts from the 90s, but I know I've gone as far as I can go with them. I thank my workouts for what they've done as I move on to something new.

What are your **Let's Do Better With This** areas?

To stop drinking soda?
To not drink with meals?
To pay attention to emotional eating?
To limit or eliminate alcohol?
To start counting protein grams?
To find a workout buddy?
To get to a support group meeting?

You owe it to yourself to take the time and think about where you can make improvements in your weight loss surgery journey. You only get one, so make it the best!

> **"When you know better, you do better."**
> **-Maya Angelou**

- 28 -

Teach It
January 28

When I saw the topic of Dr. Oz's upcoming show was about Bariatric Surgery, my first thought was, "Oh boy, here we go again. More weight loss surgery bashing."

Most television programs, commentators, and talk-show hosts, focus on the negatives of weight loss surgery. Not just complications that barely even exist anymore, but they really seem to be saying that weight loss surgery is the EASY WAY OUT. And I'm so tired of hearing it. I was tired of hearing it long before I even had weight loss surgery myself.

About ten years ago, I used to speak with people who were thinking about having surgery. At that time, weight loss surgery was not as prevalent. Consider this, between 1998 - 2002 there were just over 70,000 bariatric surgery procedures performed. But in the year 2011 alone, there were more than 158,000 of us having weight loss surgery.

Back in the early 2000s, I'd hear comments like, "My husband says I should be able to do this myself. He says he's scared about what could happen to me during the surgery." Well, we had answers for these comments. You see, by 2002, bariatric surgeons, most notably Dr. Walter Pories, had already determined that, "Gastric Bypass Cures Diabetes." So I'd say to the woman with the distressed husband, "If you needed to have a heart bypass, would your husband say the same thing?" She'd answer, "No," because most people are familiar with a heart bypass. But people didn't have the same opinion about a gastric bypass.

The media didn't help the situation much. Of course there were some positive stories and even some celebrities who had weight loss surgery. I was involved with one of those celebrities while at a previous weight loss surgery practice. I coordinated all her privacy issues and even guarded her hospital room door. I was also the liaison for CBS when they came to film a story about a young patient having weight loss surgery. The story was good and the outcome was positive. But overall, it's more interesting to run the scary weight loss surgery stories. Well, I don't know if it's because the scary stories are now fewer and further between, or because there's so much evidence out there that demonstrates how well weight loss surgery works, but the media finally seems to be giving us a break.

So, back to Dr. Oz.

When I finally saw the complete title, "The Most Underperformed Surgery in America," I thought, "What? WOW!" Specifically, the show was about the gastric bypass, because in most cases it cures diabetes. He hosted a bariatric physician and a bariatric surgeon who was also a weight loss surgery patient. They discussed all the benefits. Dr. Oz reminded the audience that this is still surgery, that the stomach and intestines were not intended to be moved around like this. But as he continued to review the improvements in a patient's health only 5 days after gastric bypass surgery, he said he was amazed at the results and was a believer.

Hallelujah!

When Dr. Oz opened the show, he said there were people in the audience who were considering weight loss surgery. At the end of the segment he asked for a show of hands, "How many are now seriously considering having the surgery because of the information you learned today?" 85% of the group raised their hands. Dr. Oz emphasized the facts he'd just provided were simple and well documented. He said the medical profession is under-informing and under-educating their patients about weight loss surgery.

How can we help as weight loss surgery patients?

First, we must remain very focused on our own daily habits of nutrition, exercise, vitamins and supplements. But we should also make an effort to educate.

Do you let others know you've had weight loss surgery or are in the process of preparing for it?

Do you understand how your surgery is performed, how the anatomy is altered during the surgery?

Do you know it well enough to explain it to someone who's thinking about it?

Do you understand the nutrition guidelines?

Do you know why you need to consume protein first?

Do you know why you need to take vitamins and supplements for life?

Do you have your exercise routine in place, so that you're able to give recommendations to someone who is just getting ready for surgery?

I really believe we owe it to our weight loss surgery brothers and sisters, pre and post, to educate them. If you knew of an amazing new cancer treatment that your neighbor just received, wouldn't you owe it to your brother with colon-cancer to share it with him?

You wouldn't think twice. You'd just do it.

Yet I know obesity is a sensitive subject. Consider coming from a perspective of sharing your personal experience instead of, "You should do what I did." Share what a difference weight loss surgery has made in your life.

Share your knowledge.

And not just with your family, friends and coworkers, but how about your physicians? Your doctor knows you've lost weight and that you're either off of or have reduced your medications, but does he know how incredible you feel? Does she know that you just had the courage to ask for a promotion and you got it? Does your doctor's office staff know you're wearing jeans you haven't worn in ten years?

If you can, please open up and talk about it. It gets easier, trust me. And it does something important for you too. It reinforces your commitment to your weight loss surgery. It reminds you how far you've come and that you want to maintain your newfound health for the rest of your life. It prompts you to make sure you've got enough vitamins and protein powder on-hand. It motivates you to exercise after work.

They say if you want to really learn something, teach it.
This is true for weight loss surgery.
So get out there and teach it.

You'll be helping yourself along the way.

- 29 -

Human Nature
February 10

We all know there are so many things that contribute to developing obesity. And perhaps many more that contribute to the development of morbid obesity.

Last weekend I enjoyed being with friends I hadn't seen in months, and some in over a year. No, this story isn't about how people reacted to my weight loss...so keep reading.

My friend Gloria has been steadily gaining about ten pounds each year, but over the last year she's gained much more and is now nearing morbid obesity. Gloria is beautiful, with sparkling blue eyes and curly, dark brown hair. She's straightforward, smart and witty. But all that seemed to be lost when she walked into the room with Leah, who's been steadily losing weight over the past few years. She's very slim now. Her clothing is stylish, her haircut and color are very current, and she was obviously feeling good about it all because she was beaming!

And truly, I'm happy for Leah.

Both women are married and seem to enjoy their careers.

Here's what I observed:

After Gloria's initial hellos, she retreated to a corner of the party and got up only to visit the buffet, get a drink or visit the bathroom. In contrast, Leah hardly sat down. She circled the room visiting with everyone. I remember when Gloria used to enjoy parties this way too.

Friends eventually made their way to Gloria's table. The conversations I overheard were, "How are you?" and "How's work?" Her responses were brief and to the point, almost as if she didn't want to engage. These aren't the conversations I remember Gloria having just a couple years ago.

But Leah was a people-magnet! I swear she had a mini crowd following her around. She's always been pleasant, sweet and friendly, but there was something different now. People were drawn to her vitality, beauty and health. And it appeared that her self-confidence had sky-rocketed because she was talking up a storm, like I'd never seen before.

At the end of the day, Gloria, Leah and I were saying farewell to our hosts, Margaret and Evelyn, the senior members of our group, each about 70-75 years. Keep in mind we've all known one other for at least two decades. Margaret and Evelyn said quick good-byes to Gloria, "It was good to see you." and "Take care Hun." It was almost like they couldn't say good-bye fast enough, almost like they were moving her along so they could get to Leah. "Oh darling! You look amazing! Incredible! You light up the room! Things must be going so well for you!" Their bodies, facial expressions and voices transformed in Leah's glow. And this was all within eye and ear-shot of Gloria.

I've learned so much about people's reactions to obesity. I guess they're just doing what comes naturally. They're drawn to beauty, to the sparkle. I suppose it's human nature.

> **"Human nature is what we were put on this earth to rise above." -The African Queen**

But my heart broke for Gloria. I understand her struggle with weight and I understand her pain, but only part of it. Because for each of us, the root of our obesity is personal. Wherever it came from and whatever continues to sustain obesity, there's pain. And so we eat, but that only takes the pain away for a few minutes, and then we have even more pain.

With weight loss surgery we have an incredible tool for weight reduction. Although not easy, following the basic guidelines leads to substantial weight loss. But make no mistake, pain and the causes of our pain don't disappear along with the pounds and the inches. The pain is something that must be addressed. And it's not just once, but over and over again that we must acknowledge what led to our obesity and caused us to stay obese.

It took me months into my post-op journey to even admit that my overeating was emotional, my way of coping. And when life gets rough, a little or a lot, there are days when I still want to turn to food to numb the pain. And honestly, there are times I have. Fortunately, I can't eat as much or eat the same foods I did before. I've been working a lot on the pain.

Why?
When?
Who?
What?
How?

This reminds me to seek out alternate ways of coping with challenging moments, and my coping options continue to grow.

- A 5-minute walk to my favorite music, away from work or home.
- A one-minute 'Tropical Vacation', courtesy of an app on my iPhone.
- Watching the latest video of my granddaughter dancing on the beach.
- Listening to my daughter sing one of her favorite songs.
- Watching a clip from one of my favorite shows like "Modern Family," "Raising Hope," or "Frasier."

Oooooooooohhhh, this is SO a daily journey. There's much

work to be done, lessons to learn and opportunities to grow. I wish you all the best, wherever you are along your journey.

> **"Face your pain, do not avoid it, breathe into it, learn from it, do not try to get rid of it, embrace it." -Jon Kabat-Zinn**

My friends' names and some details were changed in this story to protect privacy.

- 30 -

I Stopped Exercising
February 16

When there's a lot going on and life is even busier than usual, it can be any one of the important post-op guidelines that falls through the cracks like nutritious eating, adequate protein, vitamins, sleep, water or exercise. Very often, exercise can be the most challenging step. Oh my gosh, not challenging, but really hard!

We have to eat, vitamins can be kept in your purse, desk or nightstand, and sleep? Well, eventually our bodies will make us rest. But exercise…this takes time, planning and focused effort.

For the most part since surgery, I've been consistent with exercise. A day missed or skipped here and there, but overall I'm consistent. About a month ago I decided that my usual exercise routine wasn't getting me any further with my body and a change was needed. So I chose a new workout and announced it to friends, family and even at support group. With my new workout I'm watching a video with an instructor. Years ago I exercised with Jane Fonda, Kathy Smith, Karen Voight, and even Billy Blanks. My new video-instructor is pleasant, informative and encouraging. The exercise is challenging and I can feel muscles I haven't felt in a while. During the first two weeks I did the workout seven times. The third week I did it twice.

Last week, not only did I not do my new workout at all, but I couldn't bring myself to do any exercise for five days straight.

I felt defeated that I didn't keep up with the new workout, and even worse that I wasn't exercising at all.

So I set the Saturday morning alarm for 7:00 am. When it went off I woke up, looked at the time and asked myself, "why is my alarm going off at this hour on a Saturday morning?" And then I remembered why, "Oh. I'm working out this morning."

So I got dressed. I didn't head to the living room to turn on the new video, but instead headed outside with my iPhone, tuned to a new audiobook I've been looking forward to listening to, and made my way to my beloved stairs at the school near my home.

I went up and down the stairs for over an hour and I loved it. I did the same thing on Sunday but I added some of the 'new video workout' exercises to my evening routine, while watching a movie with my daughter. I also exercised Monday, and yesterday.

I've exercised 4 days in a row now.

I'm thinking about the new workout video. Was it too much? It's harder no doubt, but I know it was targeting places that my regular workout didn't. I was surprised that I could even do that workout. Intellectually, I know I need to concentrate on the new workout to get the results I want. So what's holding me back? That I won't be able to keep it up and I'll fail? Well, I've mulled this over for the last few days.

My free time, the ONLY time that's just for me, is spent exercising.

I'd say this is probably the case for many people, especially working moms. When you work, have a family, and a home to maintain, there isn't a lot of 'me' time. The 45-60 minutes I take to exercise is my 'me' time. This is why I've also used the time to listen to an audiobook, a podcast, or watch a favorite movie while I exercise. The new workout didn't allow for that. I was watching an instructor.

So here's where I am now.

I'm not making this an all or nothing. I enjoy the new workout and I know I need to do it. But right now, I can't make it the only way I spend my 'me' time. I missed being outside, and I missed my audio entertainment. For now, I'll combine the two; the effectiveness of the new workout, and the comfort of the old. I'll see how far this will take me, and then I'll make new adjustments.

After all, that's what this weight loss surgery journey and life are all about, right?

Take action.
Assess the results.
Make adjustments.
Keep going.

We got this!

- 31 -

Who's In Your Circle?
February 28

My friend said to me recently, "Now I exercise every day. I look at the gym schedule and one way or another I figure out how I'll make it to the classes. Exercise is very important to me now. I feel like it's my contribution to this thing. The surgery does what it does, and I need to do what I need to do. But I've got some friends telling me I'm addicted to exercise. These are the same people who told me not to have surgery, that I was taking the easy way out. Now they're telling me I've traded one addiction for another. Food for exercise. They don't get it."

Why is my friend's commitment to consistent exercise now considered an addiction? I bet his friends know somebody who's been at a healthy weight all their life, and they probably exercise regularly. But I bet they don't look at that person as having an addiction, they're just looked at as healthy.

A couple posts ago, I wrote about Human Nature. And here it is again.

My friend, like all of us, has stress in his life. Before surgery he ate to calm himself down, when he was sad, lonely, or even bored. But now he doesn't do that. He's embraced daily exercise and loves it. He enjoys many types of exercise, from golf to classes at the gym. A great example of the other side of Human Nature is making the best of change. My friend is living with a new situation in his life-his weight loss surgery, and he's finding ways to live with his 'new normal'.

His friends continue to judge him and his choices, and apparently think they know how to manage his life better than he does, and they have no problem telling him. More than one year after surgery, he continues to demonstrate courage and determination with healthy eating, exercise and lifestyle management. He's almost at goal weight and says he's in the process of reshaping his body. To meet his goals, he's committed to working out six days each week. And for this, he's criticized by those he cares about, by those who say they care about him. "You're addicted."

They do care about him though, right? Sometimes how we show people we care about them is really more about what we need, what we're feeling about ourselves, more so than what the person we care about needs. Ultimately, we hope his friends want the best for him, that he continues his journey toward lifelong health, and for him to be happy.

If you've already had surgery, you know firsthand this is

not the easy way out of obesity. If you're in the process of preparing for surgery, you also know this because there's so much work to do before you ever get to the operating room.

Weight loss surgery critics will most likely continue to find fault with our method. They'll find something wrong with the way we've decided to improve our health. And at some point, we must find the courage to raise our heads, look them in the eyes and tell them, "this was my choice, this is my life and my health. I am the only one who has to live in this body. And this is how I chose to improve my life." But of course, you've got to believe it yourself, first.

Do you believe it?
Are you committed to it?
Were you more committed to it one month after surgery than you are now?
What can you do to reinforce your commitment?

I went to my surgeon's support group meeting last week. Remember I'm not only a patient, I still work in this field. I work with weight loss surgery patients, developing education and preparing them for surgery. So I'm constantly reminded of all the things that are important to be successful after surgery.

ATTENDING SUPPORT GROUP IS SO IMPORTANT.

When you're in a room with 40+ people who have histories very similar to yours, and you've all made the same decision to improve your health the same way, it's wonderful. The meeting only lasted one hour but it felt so good. It was empowering. It reinforced in me again why I chose to have weight loss surgery. Hearing it stated in different ways from other weight loss surgery patients reminded me of things I hadn't thought about in a while. I wanted to cheer for them and their strength, and I did! I wanted to go up to them and say, "You keep going! You're awesome!" And I did!

Where are you getting your support?
Who is really supporting you?
The people who were supporting you before and right after surgery may be busy with other things now.
Do you feel unsupported?

If you've reached or are near your goal weight, have your friends and family stopped talking to you about it because they think your journey is over? Re-engage with those who really support you and your choices. And if those people don't exist within your immediate circle reach outside of that circle to your fellow weight loss surgery patients. We're here! Either the support group with your surgeon or a local support group, or an on-line support group. Find your circle of support. It will help you, it really will.

- 32 -

You're Building a House
March 7

> "Most people come equipped by nature with all of the pieces of a puzzle necessary to enjoy life with excellent health but by the time they get their career and family underway, most have not only managed to scramble the puzzle...they've actually lost some of the pieces" -Diane McLaren

love chance-meetings, and last night I happened upon a great one!

While leaving the local hospital I noticed the weight loss surgery support group meeting taking place in the conference room. Although the meeting had officially ended based upon the sign, there were still people in the conference room. I stepped in and asked if I could sit in for the remainder of the meeting. I was warmly welcomed by the group of about ten remaining patients. At this point, they were sharing low sugar recipes for pudding, popsicles, flavored yogurt, muffins, and smoothies.

I asked the woman with so many great low-sugar ideas, "How far out are you from surgery?" She was three years post-op. I wanted to know because I was struck by her enthusiasm for healthy food shopping, planning and preparation. She had so many great ideas. The fact that she was three years out and STILL so passionate about new recipes and maintaining a healthy diet, was inspirational.

The next motivational boost came when I asked about the lovely plate of muffins sitting in the middle of the table. A sweet woman announced she made them for the group and brought copies of the recipe for everyone. "How far out are you from surgery?" She had surgery six years ago! WOW! That's what I needed to hear, see, and really take in. There she was, LIVE and IN-PERSON, proof that the surgery works long-term and attending support group regularly is a big factor.

Most of us, when we first considered having weight loss surgery, did a lot of research. And what we learned was that weight loss surgery is effective. That's why we did it! There are so many studies that showed us for the long-haul, weight loss surgery was the answer to control our weight and rid ourselves of medical issues.

GREAT!

But tell me why so many of us choose to ignore the rest of what's in the weight loss surgery outcome studies?

You know, the studies that have followed SUCCESSFUL patients over years and years, clearly demonstrating what the keys to long-term success are. Why don't we acknowledge those success factors?

Ahhhh, there it is again. Human Nature.

Talking with fellow weight loss surgery patients, we all agree that having the actual surgery wasn't easy, but it wasn't terribly difficult either. The work comes with following the guidelines after surgery. Intellectually, we know what we have to do for maximum results, but **really** most of us knew what to do before surgery. However, we needed the surgery to serve as our catalyst for lifestyle changes. In other words, we needed something to happen to cause us to make changes.

For me, being diagnosed with Rheumatoid Arthritis, worsened by obesity, wasn't enough. Being diagnosed with diabetes type 2, wasn't enough. Being diagnosed with Hashimoto's Disease, wasn't enough. Feeling sad and discouraged everyday about my weight and about my life, was not enough to make all the lifestyle changes I needed to reduce my weight dramatically. I needed weight loss surgery.

But I'm reminded throughout each day, every day, that weight loss surgery alone isn't enough to get me where I need to go, and stay.

A great metaphor for rebuilding our health is found in **building a house**.

Think about the tools used when building a house. A hammer, tape measure, saw, level, wrench, screw driver. And the supplies. Nails, screws, wood, staples, cement, and mortar. Leave one of these tools out, and there will be BIG problems building the house. Miss one of these key supplies, and the house will be unstable.

And so it is with weight loss surgery.

It's my responsibility to make sure my weight loss surgery can utilize all the 'tools' and 'supplies' to make my health the best it can be. If I leave something out like support, a part of my long-term success is diminished. If I leave out exercise, my success is diminished. If I leave out vitamins, my success is diminished...my house is unstable.

I remember being in my Orthodontist's office when I was in grade school, and reading over and over again the prominent sign on the wall, "You don't have to floss all your teeth, just the ones you want to keep." Needless to say, I'm pretty dedicated to flossing.

So which benefits of weight loss surgery do you want to keep? All of them, right?

Great! Then learn how to use ALL the tools and supplies, so that your house - your weight loss surgery, is sturdy and strong.

"Within each of us, nature has provided all the pieces necessary to achieve exceptional health and wellness, then left it us to us to put them all together." -Diane McLaren

- 33 -

The Phantom of Fat
March 15

Phantom: Noun. A Ghost. A figment of the imagination.

Is the Phantom of Fat haunting your life?

There's a medical condition called "Phantom Limb" or "Phantom Pain." Previously, I worked in the field of Pain Management and had a few patients with this condition. Many patients with Phantom Limb pain had a limb amputated, but they still feel pain in the missing limb. What's the simplest explanation as to why they feel pain in a limb that isn't there anymore?

The brain remembers.

How does this apply to us as weight loss surgery patients?

Many of us suffer from THE PHANTOM of FAT.

Researchers have based the "Phantom of Fat" theory on the "Phantom Limb Pain" medical condition. We know firsthand what psychologists are talking about. It takes time to get used to a new body, this new size. When one has spent a significant amount of her life overweight, obese and morbidly obese - and then transforms to 'normal' in as little as a year, YES...it is difficult, even scary.

How does the PHANTOM of FAT haunt your life?

- Do you have a hard time giving away your 'big' clothes?
- Are you wearing clothes that are a couple of sizes too big?
- Do you avoid shopping for new clothes?
- When you go shopping, do you look through racks of clothes you know are too big for you?
- Have you avoided new activities, ones you thought you'd enjoy after surgery?
- Have you continued to avoid the same activities you did when you were obese?
- Do you look at yourself in the mirror and still think, or even worse - say to yourself, "I'm fat!"
- Do you say to yourself, "I may not be as fat as I was, but I'm not good enough yet because I'm not the weight / shape / size I want to be yet, so I'm still a failure."?
- Are you so afraid of gaining the weight again, so sure you're going to fail, that you won't allow yourself to enjoy the success you've achieved?
- Are you afraid to believe that this healthy weight is your new normal?
- Do you refuse to accept compliments or congratulations because you don't think you deserve them?

You can probably come up with many more ways that the PHANTOM haunts you. And why do we allow it?

Because the brain remembers.

We have so many memories, hurts, sorrows, and failures, all associated with our lives of obesity. And perhaps we occasionally used our obesity to protect us from people, activities, experiences and life. Sometimes it seems like the greater work after weight loss surgery is not exercising, eating right or taking supplements, but working on what's inside. Healing everything we've associated with obesity and making peace with our past lives. And now, accepting and making peace with our new lives in these healthier bodies.

- How long will you allow the PHANTOM of FAT to rob you of enjoying your healthier life?
- What steps can you take to reclaim your life and all that you've worked for?
- What can you do to accept that obesity is part of your past life, and that it's okay to let it go and move on?

Everything worth achieving in life takes effort, and so it is with weight loss surgery. Managing our lifestyles and healing our pasts, is all part of it. Make the effort, take the time, heal yourself.

Tell the Phantom of Fat...goodbye.

"Our deepest fear is not that we are inadequate. Our deepest fear is that we are powerful beyond measure. It is our light, not our darkness that most frightens us. We ask ourselves, 'Who am I to be brilliant, gorgeous, talented, fabulous?' Actually, who are you not to be? You are a child of God. Your playing small does not serve the world. There is nothing enlightened about shrinking so that other people won't feel insecure around you. We are all meant to shine, as children do. We were born to make manifest the glory of God that is within us. It's not just in some of us; it's in everyone. And as we let our own light shine, we unconsciously give other people permission to do the same. As we are liberated from our own fear, our presence automatically liberates others."
-Marianne Williamson

- 34 -

I Can't Eat All This
March 20

Why am I still serving myself so much? Granted, it's not the amount I served myself before surgery but it's still more than I can eat. My teenage son laughs when he sees my dinner plate, "Mom, do you really think you're going to eat all that?" Sometimes I answer him emphatically, "YES!" knowing there's no possible way I can. But my son counts on me not eating all of it so he can finish my plate. Oh the metabolism of teenage boys!

So I've checked in with some of my fellow weight loss surgery friends and asked them if they ever serve themselves too much. This is what I'm hearing back.

"It's during that transition time, the first 6 months or so after surgery, when it takes time to get used to how much you can eat."

"I think I served myself more than I could eat because I

didn't want to deny myself. I never ate it all though. I couldn't."

"I didn't want anybody else telling me how much I could eat. I think it's because I've felt that way my whole life, even when I was a child. My parents always had me on a diet. Then I put myself on stupid diets as I got older. With the surgery, I wanted to make the decision for myself how much I would serve. When I felt that I wasn't hungry enough for a large amount, then I would serve myself smaller portions. I changed my serving plate when I was ready and not before. It sounds kind of stupid, but I had to limit the amount on my plate when I was ready."

"We serve too much because that's what we've always done. We ate more than we needed to and it's a hard habit to break."

Oh my weight loss surgery friends, you've taken the words right out of my mouth!

Habits are difficult to change when you've had them for nearly all your life. And yes, I think it's Human Nature that we don't like others to put restrictions on us. If we've struggled with overweight and obesity since childhood, these feelings remind us of childhood struggles. Finally, I think it comes down to 'everything in its own time'. If we're not eating all the food we serve ourselves, and we're able to stop when we feel satisfied, then maybe there is something to be said for transitioning into the appropriate serving size when we're ready.

I actually started writing about serving myself too much three months ago. I was really struggling at that time with portion sizes. Now it's much more under control. I really am more comfortable serving myself only what I can eat. I don't feel like I'm denying myself anymore. I think it's because I've had more time to deal with the issues surrounding my obesity and my weight loss, my issues with food, and what they've been about. I'm okay with my small serving of food.

I'm okay.

- 35 -

Good Stuff, Bad Stuff...Off Track
March 27

> **"It's not what happens to you, but how you react to it that matters." -Epictetus**

Usually we talk about getting 'back on track', implying we're already 'off track'. But just in case we're doing okay, what are the warning signs we should be aware of when DANGER IS NEAR?

Going 'off track' can actually begin with something wonderful like getting to spend more time with your teenage daughter or a welcomed visit from your brother. Or it can begin with stress at work or going through a difficult breakup.

"I was exercising 4-5 days per week, for at least 45 minutes. I felt good about it and was proud that at 9-months post-op I was keeping it up. And then my daughter landed a role in her school's musical. She was thrilled and asked me to be the cast mom. I was thrilled! But this meant spending 2-3 nights per week at school. Over a period of eight weeks my exercise routine went from 4-5 days per week, to 2-3. By the time the show was over, I was down to 1 or 2 days per week. Trying to get back to your routine after that is hard. I'm still not back on track."

"My brother came to visit from England and stayed for one month. It was wonderful since I hadn't seen him in years. But he wasn't keen on having protein shakes for breakfast every day. So I started making home-style breakfasts every morning. I told myself that after he left I would get back to my morning protein shake. He's been gone six weeks and I'm still not back on track."

"There were two people at work out on medical leave. The pressure it put on me was incredible. My workday went from 9 to 12 hours a day. That crazy schedule lasted about seven weeks. But even though I'm back to 9 hours, I'm not back to my regular workout schedule. I fell back into some bad eating habits during that time too. I started eating stuff I shouldn't have to help with stress. I've gained at least 10 pounds and I'm worried I won't be able to get it off and that I'll keep gaining!"

"My girlfriend was supportive of my decision to have surgery. My surgery went well and the following 6 months were trouble free. But she seemed different. When we finally talked about it she said I was different. Yeah, I probably was different. I think I just felt better about everything. But she said it was happening too fast for her. After three years together, it was over. I used food to get through it. I couldn't eat as much but I wasn't sticking to the plan. I didn't gain weight but I wasn't losing. I've come too far and given up too much to not have this work."

And my friend, that's how it starts.

Good stuff happens and you go off track. Bad stuff happens and you go off track. Some things in life you can plan for or you know they're coming like visiting relatives or the holidays. But some things you don't see coming like being short-staffed at work, a family member becoming ill, or a relationship ending.

For the things you know are coming, get ready early. It's like preparing for the craziness of the holidays. Most of us LOVE that special time of year but we know it means life gets really busy. Develop a back-up plan for life's unanticipated events too. Either way it's life, and the key is to be realistic.

- If you can't complete your regular 45-minute workout, it's okay to opt for 20 minutes.
- If you don't have time to prepare your Tuesday night grilled chicken and steamed asparagus, opt for a similarly prepared frozen version (check nutrition facts).
- Keep high protein snacks readily available.
- Keep a resistance band with you and when you have a few minutes, stretch.

It doesn't have to be all or nothing. That's what really throws us 'off track'.

And consistent, ongoing support is critical. It's like insurance. You don't really think about it until you need it. But when you DO need it, it's there. Make it a priority to either get to a support group meeting, join an on-line support group, or develop your own group of supportive friends and family…and they don't have to all be weight loss surgery patients! This way, when you need their help and support it will already be in place.

And exercise, even in small doses, will do more than keep you in shape. It does something for you mentally. In stressful times it can remind you that there are always areas of your life where you do have control. Exercise will help you manage the stress in your life, whether it be happy stress or unpleasant, unwelcomed stress.

It was a big decision to have weight loss surgery. We owe it to ourselves, like all of the important things in life, to put effort into our backup plans. When life gets stressful, AND IT WILL, we'll be ready and not thrown off the track!

All the best with your plans.

- 36 -

My Doctor Can't See It
April 5

I had a check-up with my doctor this week. We've never met, which means she doesn't know what I looked like a year ago.

Generally speaking, primary care offices don't take pictures of their patients at every visit the way they take your blood pressure and temperature. But maybe they should.

They say a picture is worth a thousand words.

But I wonder if a picture would really help my doctor understand the full impact of weight loss surgery in my life. If she had my before and after pictures along with my medical records, would that show her everything that's changed for me?

My latest lab results tell my doctor that my blood sugars have normalized, my cholesterol levels are healthy, and my liver is no longer suffering. With the exception of low iron, which I'm working on, she can see my health has improved dramatically over the last 10 months.

But what can't she see?

My new doctor can't see what else has happened. You know, the other stuff on the inside you can't scan or run a test on.

Only I can see that. Only I can feel that.

My doctor can't. Either can a spouse, partner, parent, sister, girlfriend, boyfriend, or best friend. Even when you try to explain what you're feeling, thinking and how you've changed, you're the only one who really knows how much. I'm the only one who knows to what degree I've changed my thinking, reacting, my self-talk. I'm the only one who's aware of every thought I have and every decision I make. Only I know if I'm really eating and exercising the way I should. And when I don't, only I know the reason why…and that's only if I pay attention to the WHY.

I remember being on Weight Watchers in the early 90s. I got bored with the program and pretty much decided to starve myself Monday through Friday before my weigh-in on Saturday mornings. I'd lose 2-3 pounds then eat whatever I wanted the rest of the weekend. Monday morning, I was back to starving myself.

And guess what? It worked! I lost 80 pounds!

Everyone congratulated me on a job well done. But I knew what I was doing was crazy, and that weight loss wouldn't be sustainable. My doctor even congratulated me on my healthy eating and exercise habits after in impressive 80-pound weight loss. If only he had known the truth.

But I knew.

Ultimately, we're the doctors of our inner-selves. If we want to be healthy on the inside, we schedule the check-ups on how we're doing with things. We run the tests to see if we're utilizing the right skills for the right life situations. With these exams and results, we're able to determine if a change is needed. And when it is, we're the ones to determine what the prescription should be. It could be something basic like not buying the cookies so they aren't in the house when we're stressed, or seeking help from a therapist for Cross-Addiction.

Are you ready for this?

Weight loss surgery is a crazy journey! And like all journeys, there are forks in the road, directions to choose, decisions to make. We consult our internal-GPS and move forward with the information we have. If we're off course, if the path isn't getting us where we want to be, then we need to make a new choice.

I wish you well on your journey, as I continue with mine.

- 37 -

I Finally Took the Good Advice
April 10

I'm lucky to know many successful patients who are years out from weight loss surgery. I work with them professionally, talk with them online, and get together with them over iced tea. I love listening to their experiences and tools for success. But I find I'm one of those people, maybe like you, who has to hear the message again and again before I take the good advice.

There's a very successful patient I've known since she was in pre-op. And since surgery, I've admired her dedication to health and the way she embraces her new vitality. She's shared on more than one occasion, that the key to sticking with her daily plan is placing her before and after pictures in a prominent place in her home. Every morning and every night she looks at her before-self and current-self, and says this is all she needs to remain faithful to her nutrition, exercise, vitamins, and lifestyle changes.

"My life is whole now. The before pictures remind me to what extent my weight had limited my life. The after pictures remind me how my life has opened up. I am now completely and wholly, myself."

This wonderful patient has spoken these words to groups, she's written them down and said them to me personally. Still, it wasn't until a few days ago that I realized I hadn't taken her advice to heart. I heard her, it sounded great, but I didn't take action.

So this past weekend, I looked for 'before' pictures of myself, and like many weight loss surgery patients, there weren't too many to choose from. One of them was in my hospital gown just before surgery. And then I chose a few 'almost-after' pictures, which there aren't too many of either. I think I'm so accustomed to not wanting to see myself in pictures, and even though I'm much happier with the way I look now, I haven't translated that into getting in front of the camera. Pair that with the fact that I'm like most moms who want to capture their kids first and foremost, and the result is only a few pictures of mom! But I pulled the mini collage together and now it's on my fridge.

But before I put it up I looked at it, and then my kids looked at it. They said they had forgotten. My son said he's so used to the way I look now that he was near shock looking at the pictures.

But I wasn't in shock. I remember. I looked at the before pictures and I could feel it. And looking at the almost-after pictures, I can feel it now, in every way.

The pictures are up, and although it's only been a few days, I really like them there.

Thank you to ALL of my weight loss surgery patients and friends who share their stories with me, their advice, their knowledge, their accomplishments and their support. I am forever grateful.

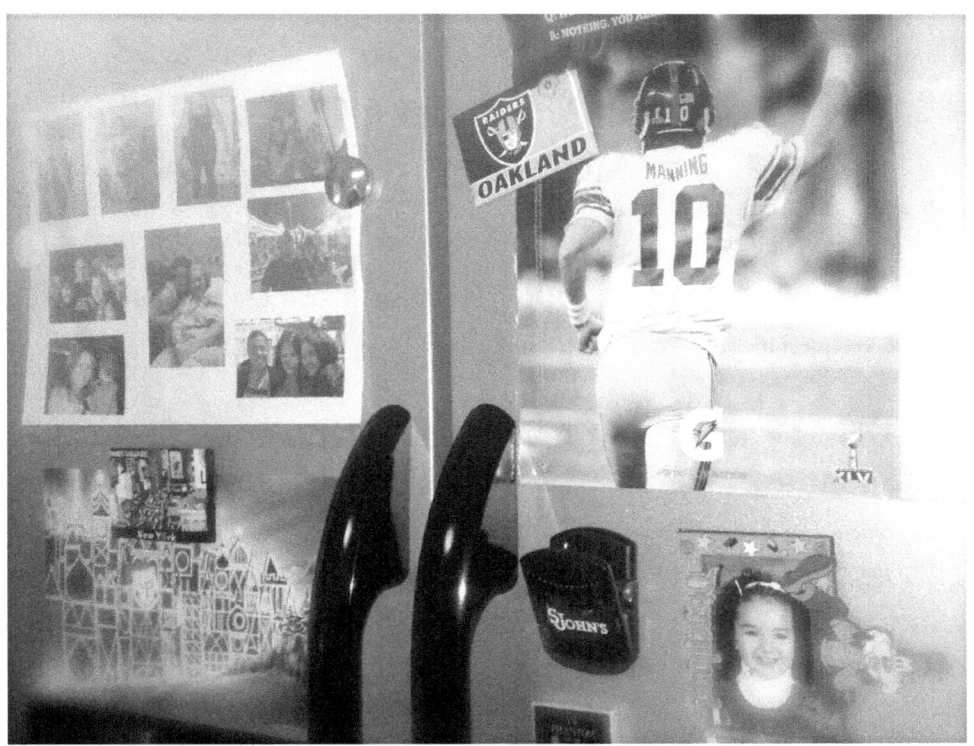

- 38 -

Come On Mom, Let's Do This
April 21

W hat works best for you? Working out by yourself, with a friend, or with a group?

What I'm hearing from my weight loss surgery friends is that most are exercising independently. Everyone's lives are so busy, it makes it difficult to pair up with a buddy and especially a group. And the few I heard from who are working out with a friend, are retired, not currently working, or exercising at work as part of a company program.

What are the benefits of working out with a friend or in a group?

ACCOUNTABILITY
"I have a hard time with motivation. We have a Monday, Wednesday, Friday arrangement at 9 am, and it's there. I schedule other things around it. I don't want to call up my buddy to reschedule. It's like I don't want to let him down."

SUPPORT

"Jen encourages me. While we're walking I talk with her about my struggles with eating, with my kids, or whatever is on my mind. She helps me with more than just my exercise. I hope I do the same for her."

STRUCTURE

"I will admit that if I wasn't walking with Jen, I may not walk as far or as long. Maybe it's because we have so much to talk about, but I walk more because of Jen!"

I workout 95% of the time, alone. With work, my kids, and running a home on my own, I have to workout around my schedule. To try and coordinate with somebody else would be hard. When I do have a partner, it's one of my kids. Last week it was my son, Adrian.

Adrian plays volleyball and is in Spring football practice. He's an athlete. So during his Easter break, I asked him to go walking with me. We headed for the half-mile hill near our home. I felt confident that I was going at a pretty good pace making my way up the hill. But I could sense that Adrian was just strolling. So I kicked it up a notch. Still, Adrian continued to stay just ahead of me with no problem. So I kicked it up again and even jogged the last part.

I made it to the top!

Coming back down though, Adrian told me about another hill around the corner. "Come on Mom, I ran up here with the team the other day. Let's do this!"

I looked at the hill and thought, "Sure. No problem." Oh boy, but it was steep! Had I been by myself, I might have said, "It's okay Mary, you already did the other hill. You don't need to go all the way to the top." Who am I kidding? I definitely would've said that.

But I was with Adrian and I wanted to keep going for myself and for him. "Come on Mom. You can make it to the white post at the top. Let's go!" I did have to stop to breathe, but then I kept going. Adrian and I stood together at the top, taking in the gorgeous sunset. What a view. Then together, we jogged back down both hills and took another quick walk around our neighborhood.

You may not be able to workout with a partner or a group consistently, but make a plan to do it once in a while. Even a couple of times a month may give you the challenge, support and encouragement you need to keep going, even stronger, even further, ever better!

Thank you, Adrian.

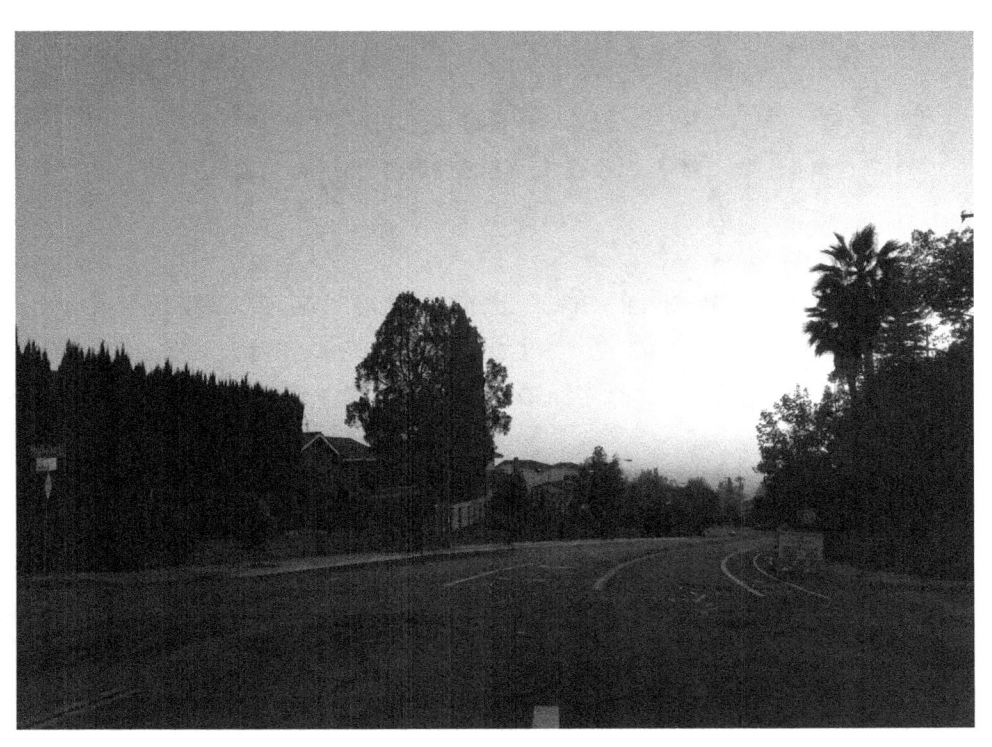

- 39 -

Back Up Plan Activated
(Or, My Son Crushed My Foot)
April 21

The same wonderful, encouraging son who inspired me to go up that second hill a couple weeks ago, stepped on my foot. Okay, he kind of crushed my foot!

Adrian wears a size 13, is about 6-feet tall and a football player. You do the math. Oh, and I didn't even have shoes on. I screamed, he jumped back, and in that instant I felt it.

PAIN!

It's five days later and the huge black and blue bruise across my foot and toes reminds me how I haven't been able to wear a shoe for the last week. I really must be thankful though. I haven't had any kind of injury since surgery that's made it difficult to exercise, and I didn't want this to be an impediment either.

The first few days I focused on more Pilates, yoga, and

strength training. But I knew the absence of cardio would start to catch up with me. I have a Jillian Michaels - Aerobic Step Deck/Balance Board. I've only used it for step aerobics so far. But a couple days ago I took off the steps and put on the balance-board disc. I'm able to use this option in bare feet. Ten minutes into the rocking, I was sweating. A few YouTube videos demonstrated some cardio-balance variations and they worked. They included 5 pound weights and resistant tubes. After 45 minutes I was sweating. My kids were surprised and so was I.

Things happen. You get tied up at work, a family member needs your help, or your football-player son with size 13 feet crushes your foot. We have to have backup plans for nutrition, exercise, and lifestyle management.

Do you have backup plans?

- 40 -

My One-Year Anniversary
May 23

Many weight loss surgery patients consider the date of their surgery as their new birthday, the day they were reborn!

But today, I will celebrate my son's birthday as the first reason to rejoice on May 23rd, and yes I'm also celebrating the second time I was wheeled into an operating room on this day. One year ago, after 10 years of seeing what weight loss surgery can do, I put my trust in an excellent surgeon and his team, and trusted myself to take charge of my health.

It was the best decision for my heath and has done more for my life over the past year than I could have ever imagined possible.

There are many people to thank for everything this surgery has been and continues to be in my life.

My surgeon, for your skill and support. You are an amazing human being and a blessing in my life.

My family, for your patience, encouragement, coaching, and unconditional love.

My friends, for being happy for me, loving me, checking on and supporting me.

To my fellow patients and weight loss surgery friends whom I've talked with in-person, online, via email, and over the phone. You're all so inspiring. Just when I think I've heard it all you give me new information, new ideas, and new ways of looking at things that get me through another challenge.

Here are some numbers that demonstrate what weight loss surgery has done in my life.

My blood pressure in April, 2011: 139 / 77
My blood pressure in April, 2012: 99 / 57

My resting heart rate in April, 2011: 76
My resting heart rate in April, 2012: 60

Other great numbers from April, 2011 to April, 2012:

LDL cholesterol (the bad one): 107 to 83

Triglycerides: 98 to 59

My surgeon took a biopsy of my liver during surgery and I was diagnosed with non-alcoholic fatty liver disease. My

ALT result (blood test for liver damage) in April, 2011 was 134. In April, 2012, my ALT result is 26!

Before surgery I wore 18-20, now I wear a medium, or an 8-10.

My BMI before surgery was 40.
My BMI today is 26.

I used to inject insulin, was on three diabetes medications, and took medications for other conditions too, making it eleven pills a day.

How many now? Two.

My conditions are auto-immune and not completely resolved, but considered in remission. For now, my physician wants to be cautious.

What about other numbers?

Before surgery, how many days did I wake up...
- Wishing I wasn't obese.
- Wondering which diet I should start.
- Praying for the strength to stick with a diet and exercise plan.
- Pleading with God to not let my diabetes or other conditions get any worse.

SEVEN days a week.

Since my surgery, how many days have I felt this way?

ZERO.

How many times do I second guess myself when I walk into a room of strangers or, let me be honest, even into a room of people I know without feeling ***not good enough***?

ZERO.

How many days do I worry about my kids being embarrassed of me when I go to their events, even though they've never said a word about it?

ZERO.

How many times do I avoid going to the doctor because I don't want to be weighed?

ZERO.

How often do I dread special events like a wedding or family reunion because I'll have to go on a starvation diet and never find the right clothes to cover up my body?

ZERO.

How many nights have I worried that my foot would eventually be amputated due to severe diabetic neuropathy?

ZERO.

How many mornings have I cried while staring at my body

in a full length mirror?

ZERO.

How many times have I spoken to myself horribly, telling myself I deserve to be uncomfortable in my tight Spanx, with deep red marks all over my stomach, because it was my fault I was so fat?

ZERO.

How many days have I hidden in my home ashamed to go anywhere unless I HAD TO?

ZERO.

There are many more ZEROs, and if you're even a few months out from weight loss surgery you probably already have your own ZERO list. You know how unbelievably amazing this new life is.

And I am grateful to God my Father for this blessing, for my renewed health, for all the opportunities that have opened up for me, and for His unceasing love and guidance.

There were times during this past year, with some serious issues going on in my family, when I wondered how I would have made it through this difficult time without my weight loss surgery. I'll tell you how I would have done it…with food. I can't even think about how much weight I would have gained by now, how much worse my diabetes would have been, how less capable I would have been to take care of my kids or even function efficiently because I would have used food to comfort and numb myself. I probably would have put on 25 pounds by now. I don't even want to think about what that would have done to my diabetes.

But here I am. Healthier, happier and hopeful.

I don't know what the next year has in store for me. I could have never seen the difficult events of the last year coming, and I'm so grateful my weight loss surgery happened when it did. I had to find alternatives to food for coping and comfort, and I have.

I've learned a lot about myself over the last year, and some of it was hard to take in. But it was the truth, and I needed to know so I can make better choices for my future.

I've also learned what I'm capable of when I need to depend on myself. I've learned again that physical exercise is just as important for my heart and mind as it is for my body…maybe even more so. I've learned that the help, the people and the resources I needed to get through tough things have been there all along…but weight loss surgery shined a light on them.

This poem is hanging in my bathroom. It describes my year. It makes me cry and smile at the same time.

> "The time will come
> when, with elation,
> you will greet yourself arriving
> at your own door, in your own mirror
> and each will smile at the other's welcome,
> and say, sit here. Eat.
> You will love again the stranger who was yourself.
> Give wine. Give bread. Give back your heart
> to itself, to the stranger who has loved you
> all your life, whom you ignored
> for another, who knows you by heart.
> Take down the love letters from the bookshelf,
> the photographs, the desperate notes,
> peel your own image from the mirror.
> Sit. Feast on your life."
> - Derek Walcott

If you're thinking about having weight loss surgery,
if you're scheduled for surgery,
if you just had surgery,
or even if you had surgery years ago...

I understand in some way where you are and where you've been. In one way or another, I have too. If I could hug you and tell you, "Thank you," and "I'm here for you," I would.

Sharing my first year after weight loss surgery has been my way of reaching out to you, relating to you, hoping that my words would help you in some way. Your generous responses to my stories, through e-mails and personal words when I've seen you in person, have helped me in so many ways.

Thank you, my friend. I appreciate you and all you've done by allowing me to share this incredible year with you.

When I began writing over a year ago, I never thought about how long this would go on. I just started typing. And now, here we are. I plan to keep writing every couple weeks and sharing my experiences during Year Two.

You know what? I just took a big breath when I thought, "I have no idea what's coming this year." It can be a little scary.

But I know I'm better equipped to handle whatever is coming because of everything I've been through, and I know I wouldn't feel this way if I didn't have my weight loss surgery.

Yes. That feels good to say.

I HAVE WEIGHT LOSS SURGERY!

And you can HAVE it too.

Love to you my friend,

Mary

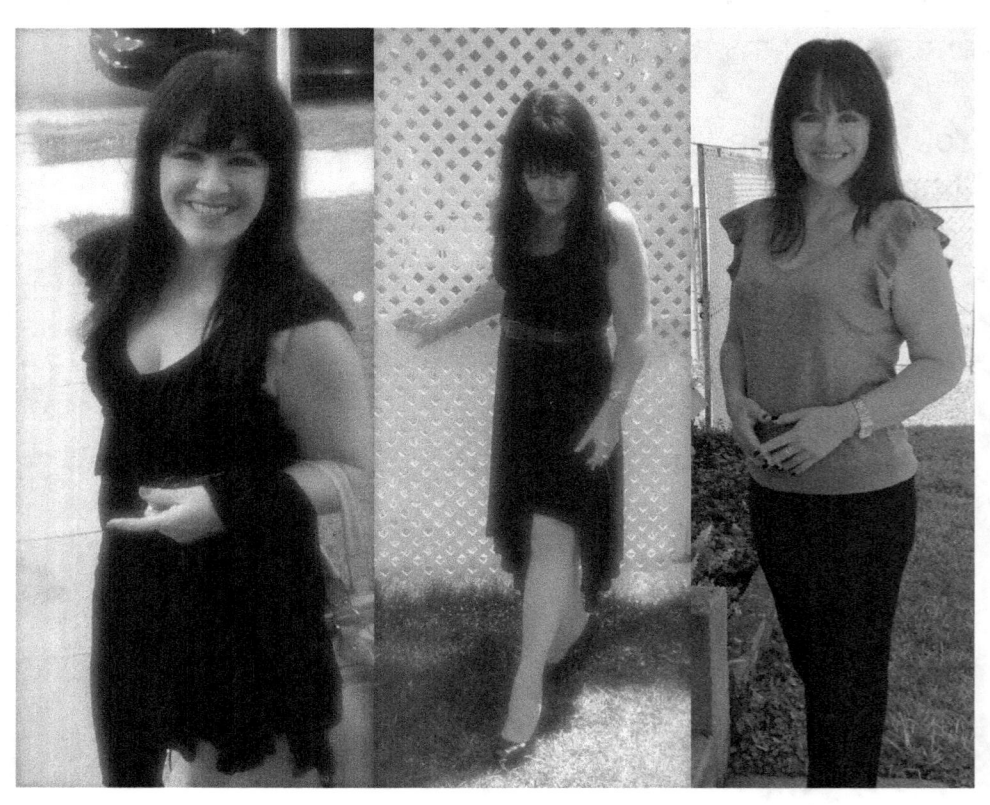

- Afterword -

Well sweetheart, that's "Year One." You may notice I never address my divorce directly. I couldn't for legal and personal reasons. Even though I was learning a lot about myself and how to take steps toward self-compassion, my head continued to spin as details that induced the breakup surfaced almost weekly.

In preparing "Year One" for you, I realized while reading each story I'd actually documented not just the first year of my life after weight loss surgery, but the first year of my emotional, mental and spiritual transformation.

But my journey had dark periods too. And now, as I'm reading through my "Year Two" stories, I'm reminded of my challenges with cross-addiction and self-image. In "Year Two," as I worked to get comfortable with my normal weight and extra skin, I faced my child's rare medical diagnosis, the challenges of solo-parenting two teenagers, my mom's death, and the ongoing divorce saga.

Yet even with all that, here I am today. Five years after weight loss surgery and nearly five years after my marriage ended, I am the happiest, healthiest and most at peace I've ever been in my life.

Sweetheart, I mean it with all my heart when I tell you I want this for you too. We'll talk again soon, when "Now It's Mary's Turn – Year Two," is released.

Until then, please make sure we're connecting through social media, email, and on nowitsmaryturn.com where you'll find more awesome resources I'm creating for you every week!

And if you haven't already, make sure to download your BONUS gift, the "Year One - Workbook." But it's not just a gift to browse through. Yes, it's pretty and has some of my favorite quotes, but sweetheart it's a workbook created to help you make the most of where you are on your weight loss surgery journey. And I'll be checking in to see how you're coming along with it, okay?

Okay!

Love, light and grace to you.

You can download your "Year One - Workbook" at nowitsmarysturn.com/activate.

www.ingramcontent.com/pod-product-compliance
Lightning Source LLC
Chambersburg PA
CBHW060311290526
45789CB00001B/478